PRINCIPLES OF
BACH FLOWER REMEDIES

other titles in the series

PRINCIPLES OF

BACH FLOWER REMEDIES

What it is, how it works and what it can do for you

Revised Edition

Stefan Ball

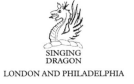

SINGING
DRAGON
LONDON AND PHILADELPHIA

This edition published in 2013
by Singing Dragon
an imprint of Jessica Kingsley Publishers
116 Pentonville Road
London N1 9JB, UK
and
400 Market Street, Suite 400
Philadelphia, PA 19106, USA

www.singingdragon.com

First published in 1999 by Thorsons, and imprint of HarperCollins
Copyright © Stefan Ball 1999 and 2013

Library of Congress Cataloging in Publication Data
A CIP catalog record for this book is available from the Library of Congress

British Library Cataloguing in Publication Data
A CIP catalogue record for this book is available from the British Library

ISBN 978 1 84819 142 6
eISBN 978 0 85701 120 6

Printed and bound in Great Britain

CONTENTS

ACKNOWLEDGEMENTS

I am grateful to Elaine Abel, Lucille Arcouet, Rosemary Barry, Claudia Belou, Barbara Davis, Elaine Hollingsworth, Ingrid Lewis and Rae Ramsey for permission to include their accounts of the remedies in action.

Thanks also to the team at The Bach Centre and in particular Judy Ramsell Howard, Kathy Nicholson, June King and Emma Broad.

I first learned about the remedies from my wife Chris in the early 1990s. My love and dedication go to her and our children, Alex, Maddie and Ethan.

Introduction

Western Medicine

The Western world's approach to dealing with health has on the whole been extremely successful. Even countries like India and China, which have very different medical traditions of their own, accept and use the West's model. But what exactly is orthodox Western medicine?

At the risk of oversimplifying, we could say that Western medicine represents a reductionist, physical approach based on the use of drugs and technology. It is reductionist because it reduces people to sets of symptoms so as to intervene at that level. It is physical because it deals almost exclusively with bodies. And the fact that it is based on drugs and technology is graphically shown by the different values placed on people and machines in modern health services: money is lavished on new drugs, machines and techniques, while nurses remain relatively underpaid.

If you have a wheeze in your chest, the doctor will start by listening to your breathing. Then he will prescribe a drug or other treatment designed to deal with the inflammation or congestion that is causing the wheeze. If the doctor asks you how you feel apart from the wheeze, you will probably understand this to relate to your physical condition. You are likely to mention a sore throat and less likely to mention that you lost your job yesterday.

This approach is very effective at dealing with physical symptoms like the wheezing chest, because drugs are tailor-made to attack the physical cause of symptoms. It is also spectacularly successful when it comes to injuries such as fractured legs, ribs and skulls. The doctor can use the technological equipment at his disposal to isolate the problem and then use physical means to repair it – straightening the leg, binding up the rib and tacking metal plates onto the skull.

Lives are saved every day using scientific Western medicine. But for many it is still failing.

People as cars

The magic bullet idea of medicine – that there is a physical solution to every physical symptom – is in turn based on a philosophical view of human life that stresses the complete separateness of our physical and mental worlds. 'I think therefore I am,' said Descartes, but the 'I' he referred to was not his stomach or his arms or his heart. Instead, 'I' is somewhere in the head. 'I' looks out through its eyes, and its body is something else – a sort of vehicle that 'I' gets carried around in. The thoughts and feelings of 'I' don't have any real effect on the body because there is no direct connection. 'I' can do what it wants with its body, as long as it gets it serviced from time to time and takes on enough fuel.

Perhaps this explains why some of us treat our bodies much the same as we treat our cars. We go too fast; we don't look after ourselves; we crash; we take ourselves off to the doctor to be fixed up. Doctors become glorified garage mechanics, replacing worn-out parts and rebuilding bits of broken machinery.

A problem with the orthodox approach

To continue the metaphor, one problem with the orthodox approach is that while the car is being repaired, the driver is often not treated at all. He sits around waiting for the vehicle to be fixed and then off he goes, driving just as badly as before, until once again he crashes.

The main criticism of the orthodox approach is that it does not do enough for that part of us that cannot be seen. The 'I' in its head is not considered, when in fact the 'I' is often the cause of the body's disease. Beyond the 'I', at the level of spirit or soul, the problem is worse. In much of modern Western medicine, the soul of the patient is not only not considered: for all practical purposes it isn't there at all.

Holistic medicine

Treat the person, not the disease. This is the holistic approach in a nutshell, and the focus on the whole person is the main difference between holism and orthodox Western medicine. Holism puts forward the view that spirit, mind and body are interconnected in countless subtle ways. Holistic medicine seeks to view and treat people in their entirety so as to address all aspects of their lives at once.

Some methods, such as reflexology and acupuncture, direct the majority of their attention to physical problems, but do so using a system that also affects the mental and spiritual side of our beings. Others seek to prescribe for both levels at once. Homoeopathy is a good example of the latter, with its mix of physical and mental symptomatology.

Working with the Bach remedies, however, means taking a third route. Diagnosis and treatment happen on the level of emotion, spirit and mind, on the theory that balance here will in turn affect the health of the body. Emotional states are used as the key to unlock the body's natural capacity to heal itself.

Psychoneuroimmunology

In many ways, the holistic approach is becoming part of the mainstream. Most doctors accept that stress and emotional imbalance contribute to anything up to 95 per cent of all disease, and there has been a flurry of research in the US into the effect of emotions on the immune system. Dr Robert Ader, working at the University of Rochester in 1975, was the first person to call this subject psychoneuroimmunology, or PNI for short.

PNI is the study of how people's states of mind influence their physical health through links between the brain and the immune system. More and more mainstream scientists now work in this area. Positive research results have appeared in major professional journals such as the UK's *The Lancet* and the US's *Proceedings of the National Academy of Sciences.*

At Ohio State University, for example, one study found that people struggling with the pressures of caring for relatives with Alzheimer's disease tended to suffer from worse colds than other people. Another showed that people with high anxiety levels had less effective protection from antibodies and immune cells.

These and other studies have demonstrated that stress leads to the release of neurotransmitters and hormones and that these in turn change cellular activity in the immune system. It seems that the immune system is equipped with receptors that can decode emotional messages from the brain.

PNI tends to confirm what holism has always claimed, that a lack of harmony in the mental or spiritual spheres will lead eventually to physical illness. A further interesting result of PNI research has been to show that people who feel in control of their lives and emotions are less likely to be sick than those who feel that they are controlled by fate, the elements or some other external force.

What are Bach flower remedies?

This is where the Bach system fits in. Bach remedies are medicines for the emotions that aim to balance negative states of mind and resolve character defects by encouraging the corresponding virtue. This means that we can all gain the health benefits of having a balanced emotional life. And because they are simple tools that anyone can learn to use, they give to every one of us the power to take control of our emotions. We can all be inner-directed, and PNI research shows that this alone can lead us to feel healthier and better about our lives.

There are 38 remedies in the system. Of these, 37 are made from a single flower or plant. The thirth-eighth is a specially prepared spring water.

Each remedy is aimed at a specific negative emotion, such as fear, lack of confidence, or worry. The remedies do not impose an effect in the way many orthodox drugs do, by damping down symptoms. Instead they enhance our existing positive qualities. The negative state is not suppressed: it is removed by an increase in the corresponding positive emotion. The result of taking the appropriate remedy is to give courage, increase confidence or quiet the worrying mind.

Bach flower remedies bring holistic healing into the hands of everyone. Dr Bach was fond of referring to them as the medicine of the future. Before growing towards that future, however, it will be helpful to look back at the roots of the system, to answer the obvious question: who was Dr Bach, and where did the remedies come from?

1

Where Do Bach Flower Remedies Come from?

Dr Edward Bach

The man who discovered the 38 remedies was called Edward Bach. ('Bach' is pronounced 'Batch', to rhyme with 'match'.) He was born in the West Midlands in 1886, where his father owned a brass foundry. When he left school he worked at the foundry for a time, but he soon left to study medicine, first at Birmingham University and later at University College Hospital in London, where he qualified in 1912.

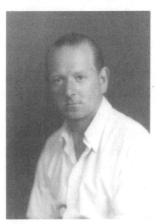

Figure 1.1 Dr Edward Bach

Trained as an orthodox doctor, Bach's career path started off in an equally orthodox manner. After qualifying he took a place as casualty medical officer at University College Hospital, and he also held the post of casualty house surgeon at the National Temperance Hospital until his own ill health obliged him to give up that position. He opened consulting rooms near Harley Street and soon became interested in immunology, leading to research work as a bacteriologist at University College Hospital.

It was here that he first began to make a name for himself as an original thinker. He was intrigued by the problem of chronic disease and by its possible relationship to certain bacteria that seemed to proliferate in the intestines of some of his patients. He produced vaccines from seven different types of bacteria and gave them to his patients. The results were extremely good.

When the First World War started in 1914 Dr Bach tried to enlist, but was turned down repeatedly because of his poor state of health. Determined to do what he could, he took on extra duties at the hospital, where he was in charge of more than 400 beds reserved for war casualties. His research work continued unabated, while his health deteriorated to such a degree that in 1917 he suffered a haemorrhage and lost consciousness.

An immediate operation was carried out to remove a cancerous growth, but the prognosis was poor. When Dr Bach came round his colleagues told him that at the very most he had three months left to live.

Dr Bach left his hospital bed as soon as he was able to walk and plunged himself back into his work. If he only had a little time, he would use it to make as great a contribution as he could and complete if possible his work on chronic disease.

He worked every hour of the day and night. He was so wrapped up in his research and war work that he hardly noticed that his strength was returning and that he had already outlived the most optimistic of his colleagues' predictions. In her biography (1940) Nora Weeks tells of one of the doctors who had treated Dr Bach returning from the front some time after the operation. He was so surprised to see Dr Bach walking around that he greeted him with the words, 'But, good God! Bach, you're dead!'

Ever since his days in the brass foundry Dr Bach had been aware that the fear of illness was as great a problem as illness itself. Workers were terrified of falling sick because it would mean the loss of income and no food on the table. The fear alone seemed to make illness more likely. Thinking now about his own miraculous recovery, he saw a link between his reaction to the diagnosis of cancer and his return to health. He became convinced that he had got better because he was too engaged with life and with his life's work to feel fear. His vocation had saved him.

Homoeopathic principles

Dr Bach's work with the bacterial vaccines was very successful, but there were some aspects of it that he found distasteful. In particular he disliked the idea of giving injections to patients.

He found a partial answer to this problem when he found that he got better results by only giving further doses of the vaccine once all improvement from the first dose had stopped. Instead of giving injections at regular intervals, the new method meant that sometimes he only had to give a repeat dose after many months.

The next breakthrough came in 1919, when Dr Bach started work as a pathologist and bacteriologist at the London Homoeopathic Hospital. Required reading for this new job was Samuel Hahnemann's seminal work *The Organon of Rational Medicine*. As he read the book, Dr Bach was startled to find that without knowing it he had been following in Hahnemann's footsteps: the founder of homoeopathy had identified the principle of the minimum dose and the link between intestinal toxaemia and chronic disease a century before. Dr Bach also felt great sympathy with the homoeopathic principle of treating people as individuals rather than concentrating on the disease alone, and with the use in some homoeopathic remedies of natural substances, including plants.

The seven Bach nosodes

It was natural for Dr Bach to wonder how other ideas contained in *The Organon of Rational Medicine* might relate to his own work. Accordingly, he tried preparing his vaccines using homoeopathic methods. The results were excellent, and as the homoeopathic vaccines were administered by mouth he was able to abandon the use of injections.

The new homoeopathic vaccines became known as the seven Bach nosodes. Along with other bowel nosodes prepared by Dr Bach's colleagues, they are still in use today.

Treating the person, not the disease

Homoeopathic medicines are not prescribed for the patient's physical symptoms alone. Practitioners also take account of the type of person being treated and of her state of mind. These non-physical symptoms are sometimes referred to as 'mentals'.

Dr Bach began to make notes on the different personalities of the people he was treating. Soon he was able to build up a picture of the mentals associated with each of the seven nosodes. As time went by he found he was able to predict which nosode a person needed from observation of his character alone. He still carried out laboratory analyses of bacterial specimens, but more and more it was only to confirm a diagnosis at which he had already arrived.

Despite these successes, Dr Bach remained less than satisfied with what he had achieved. He was making the nosodes from bacteria taken from the intestines of sick people. The nosodes were the products of disease. He disliked the idea of building health on sickness and was convinced that somewhere in nature there would be a purer type of medicine that would be wholly positive in its action.

The theory of types

Dr Bach began to collect plants and take them back to his laboratory. He prepared them using standard homoeopathic methods and compared the effects of the resulting medicines with the cures obtained using the original nosodes. Over time he found a few plants that had a similar effect to some of the nosodes, but the match was never exact.

One night Dr Bach was attending an official dinner. Out of boredom he began to observe the other guests and to divide them into groups, according to their characters and behaviour, in much the same way that he divided people into groups when selecting a nosode for them.

However, instead of only seven groups he quickly sketched out more. He wondered at first whether each of these new groups would be associated with a particular disease, but he realised that this was not so. Rather, each group of people would tend to react in the same ways to any disease that they caught.

Up to this point Dr Bach's work had only been aimed at a specific kind of chronic disease. Now he saw how the new scheme that he had begun to sketch out might lead to a truly complete system, one that would be able to treat all diseases. It would do this by treating people's basic emotional imbalances. It would represent a much greater application of the homoeopathic principle of treating the whole person.

Discovery of the flower remedies

In September 1928 Dr Bach found the first of the plants that were to form part of the system of 38 flower remedies. These were Impatiens and Mimulus, which he brought back to London from Wales, and prepared in his laboratory in the same way that he had prepared so many plants before.

He matched the plants to two of the personality groups that he had worked out and tried them on his patients. A third remedy was soon added to the first two, this time made from Clematis.

The results were so good that by the end of the following year Dr Bach had stopped using the nosodes completely. A few months later, early in 1930, he decided to leave London to devote himself full time to finding more healing plants and to developing the new system. His colleagues were stunned by his decision, but his conviction and enthusiasm were such that Dr Bach overcame all objections. By May of that year he was on his way, accompanied by a radiographer called Nora Weeks, who had agreed to go with him as his assistant.

Dr Bach spent the next four years travelling all over the southern half of Britain, from north Wales to East Anglia. He walked much of the time, constantly looking for new plants to prepare, but the first discovery he made was of a new method of preparing remedies – one that was far simpler than any in homoeopathy, and one more in keeping with his wish to find a natural medicine.

The sun method

Even before he left London Dr Bach was aware that his sensitivity towards the energy in plants had been growing. He was able to feel the resonance or vibration of a flower simply by holding it in his hands. Some would bring calm and strength, while others would cause nausea and other physical reactions.

Dr Bach discovered a new method of capturing the potency of flowers very early one sunny morning when he was walking through a field in Wales. The flowers sparkled under a layer of dew, and it occurred to him that the heat of the sun might be enough to draw their strength into the liquid, creating a natural preparation.

He decided to test out this theory, and set to work to collect dewdrops. Some he took from flowers that had been in full sunlight, the rest from plants growing in the shade. The results confirmed his intuition: there was indeed a potency in the liquid he had collected, and it was far stronger in the dew taken from the sun-warmed flowers.

The next step was to find a practical way to use this discovery. It would take too long to collect dew in sufficient quantities, so Dr Bach tried using a bowl of water instead. He collected flowers and laid them on the water in the sunlight. After a time he tested the resulting liquid, and to his delight it was just as powerful as the harvested dewdrops had been.

This method was the one that he used to prepare all of the remedies he found during his period of wandering – 19 of them in all.

Mount Vernon

By 1934, Dr Bach was looking for somewhere more permanent to live. He had always liked the Thames Valley, so when Nora Weeks found a small empty cottage called Mount

Vernon available for rent in Sotwell, just outside Wallingford, he decided to take it. Moving in, he was delighted to find that most of the 19 remedies he had already discovered grew in the countryside around his new house.

Funds were low – Dr Bach spent all he had on his work and rarely charged for help – so he built much of the furniture for the house himself, cutting and staining the wood by hand. He also threw himself into gardening. He dug out the worst of the weeds and planted wild flowers by throwing handfuls of seeds into the air. In a more orthodox fashion, he laid out lawns and used some of the rubble left by previous inhabitants to create paths.

The last 19 remedies

Dr Bach had 19 remedies already, but he had become aware of gaps in the system, and in the spring of 1935 he again began to look for new remedies.

His sensitivity at this time had developed to an alarming degree, and he suffered intensely from the negative states of mind for which he needed remedies. Often a negative emotional state would be accompanied by severe physical pain; nevertheless he would go out and look for the plant that he needed to rebalance his emotions. At this time he really was his own laboratory.

He suffered in this way all through the spring and summer of 1935. By August he had found a further 19 remedies. The system was complete: he now had a remedy for every basic negative emotion from which people could suffer.

The boiling method

The first of the new series of remedies was found in March. At this time Dr Bach was suffering from a severe sinusitis, which was accompanied by a feeling of utter desperation, as though he was losing his mind. He wanted to prepare the blossoming twigs of the cherry plum tree, which his intuition told him might hold a cure. But in March the sun would not be warm enough to potentise such tough plant material using the sun method. He needed to look for a different way to extract the healing energy.

He decided to try boiling the flowering twigs in water. Heat from a fire would replace the heat of the sun. He let the water and greenery bubble for half an hour and then left the pan outside to cool before filtering off the liquid. He took a few drops, and the desperation and pain faded at once, confirming the choice of plant and the usefulness of this new method of preparation.

The Bach Centre

Dr Bach died on 27 November 1936, a year after finding the last remedy. He left all he had to Nora Weeks and asked her and their friends Victor Bullen and Mary Tabor to continue his work and follow the principles he had set out. 'As soon as a teacher has given his work to the world, a contorted version of the same must arise,' he wrote to Victor a month before his death. 'Our work is steadfastly to adhere to the simplicity and purity of this method of healing.'[1]

Mary left the team in the 1940s, so it was Nora and Victor who carried things on, making remedies and giving consultations and advice to people who arrived at the house looking for help. The remedies were never advertised. Word of mouth and personal recommendation were what allowed news of them to spread, little by little, all over the world.

---

1   This and other quotations from Edward Bach appear in *The Original Writings of Edward Bach* (Howard and Ramsell 1990). See Further reading at the end of the book.

Supporters of their work raised the money to allow Nora and Victor to buy Mount Vernon in 1958. They set up a trust when completing the purchase so that the house and garden would remain the centre of Dr Bach's work for all time, as he had intended. Over the years the house and the people in it became known as The Bach Centre.

Victor died in 1975, and Nora three years later. But they had already made plans to pass on their responsibilities to brother and sister John Ramsell and Nickie Murray. Nickie retired from the Centre in 1988, and John's daughter Judy Ramsell Howard took her place. John passed away in 2008, leaving Judy at the head of the small team at the Centre.

Back in 1936, Dr Bach gave an address in Wallingford on his birthday. He intended it to be the first in a series of lectures aimed at spreading news of his discoveries to as many people as possible. But he died just a month later.

So when the old bottling rooms at Mount Vernon were converted into a seminar room in 1991 and the first of a series of courses held, the Centre was picking up a thread that had been left long untied. Years later, Bach Centre-approved courses are available in more than 40 countries around the world, and the register of trained practitioners held at the Centre grows every year.

Every one of those thousands of courses aims to teach the original, simple system exactly as Dr Bach left it. Education and the work of registered Bach practitioners has become the main focus of The Bach Centre's continuing promise to its founder.

How are remedies made?

One of the first times I prepared a remedy was late one summer when gentian had come into flower in one of Dr Bach's original remedy-making sites. A look at what happened that day gives a good picture of how remedy makers generally work.

The weather forecast was excellent – clear skies and sun expected all across England – so I took the necessary equipment home with me the night before. Everything was carefully wrapped to keep it clean and ready for an early start.

The morning was as lovely as had been promised. My wife Chris decided to come along for the ride. Our daughter Madeleine (just turned three at the time) had a prior engagement, so we dropped her off early before setting off for the site.

We climbed a hill to get to the flowers. Ethan, five months old, was in his backpack. Alexandra, soon to be six and enjoying her first summer holiday from school, went racing ahead.

The site used that day is on private land. There is a well-worn track to the top, which opens out suddenly giving wonderful views across the open country of the Thames valley. We reached the summit at about 8.30am. We rested for a few minutes then, with the sun getting hotter as it climbed, began to collect the flowers.

The plant used for the Gentian remedy is *Gentiana amarella*, the autumn gentian. It is a spiky, upright plant, rarely more than a foot high. A good example will be covered with purple flowers.

It is important when picking the flowers not to touch them with your hands. One approach is to hold a half-litre glass bowl in one hand, two-thirds filled with water, and snip the stalks with scissors so that the flowers drop directly onto the surface. Collecting flowers like this is painstaking work, so Chris and I did it between us, while Ethan slept and Alex looked for rabbits.

Once its surface is a little more than covered with flower heads, the bowl can be carefully topped up with more water before being placed in sunlight, away from any shade. The bowl needs to stay in unbroken sunshine for three hours. Remedy makers dread cloud, especially when it gathers in the late morning. It can mean a whole day's work has been wasted.

On this particular day we ended up with seven bowls sitting in the sun, the water twinkling in the light, refracting the blue-purple gentian flowers. There were hundreds – maybe thousands – of plants that we had not touched, but we didn't try to make more remedy. We had enough and didn't want to disturb the plants more than we had to.

To complete the process the energised water is mixed half and half with 40 per cent proof brandy and poured into one-litre brown glass medicine bottles. The bottle are given a quick shake to mix up the contents and then labelled and taken to the tincture store for safekeeping.

These concentrated, one-litre remedy mixes are called mother tinctures. They are diluted into liquid to make the stock remedies you see on sale in shops. Most often the liquid used is brandy – sometimes euphemistically referred to on the label as 'grape alcohol solution'. This was Dr Bach's preferred option and makes the traditional stock remedy. Some remedy makers mix mother tinctures into other preservatives as well, including combinations of glycerine and water, and 'denatured' alcohol with added salt. In all cases, the ratio of mother tincture to carrying liquid should be two drops to every 30 ml.

There are several companies making and selling stock remedies. Some supply them in 10 ml bottles, others in 20 ml. If you have a 10 ml bottle of remedy it should contain two-thirds of a drop of mother tincture. A 20 ml remedy bottle will contain one-and-one-third drops.

2

Who Uses Bach Flower Remedies?

On simplicity

At the end of so many years of research into so many different aspects of medicine, we might have expected that Dr Bach would leave behind shelves full of textbooks, journal articles, papers and notes – the whole only understandable after long study and a great deal of effort.

In fact he summed up his life's work in about 30 pages, in a little booklet called *The Twelve Healers and Other Remedies*. At different times in his life he destroyed his notes and papers and with them went evidence of the work that had gone into creating the system. He burned in a bonfire at Mount Vernon much of the material that might have ended up making the bookshelves groan.

He was clear about the reason for doing this. He wanted to avoid leaving behind anything that might complicate the system and make it harder for people to use. This determination comes across clearly in the introduction to the final version of *The Twelve Healers and Other Remedies*:

> This system of treatment is the most perfect which has been given to mankind within living memory. It has the power to cure disease; and, in its simplicity, it may be used in the household.

It is its simplicity, combined with its all-healing effects, that is so wonderful.

No science, no knowledge is necessary, apart from the simple methods described herein; and they who will obtain the greatest benefit from this God-sent gift will be those who keep it pure as it is; free from science, free from theories, for everything in Nature is simple.

Simplicity was one of Dr Bach's favourite words. It was the cornerstone of his approach to medicine, an approach that empowers the patient and takes power away from the expert. In the Bach system the patient does not have to remain patient. Instead she is able to grasp the system and use it to heal herself and the people around her.

Over the years people have come up with new ways of using the remedies, new approaches to selection and dosage, and new theories as to how they work. Others have recreated Dr Bach's discarded theories and used them to reinterpret his final findings. But the system Dr Bach left remains what it has always been: the most effective approach to self-help and self-healing ever discovered, the easiest to learn, and the simplest to use.

Self-healing

During the decades that have passed since Dr Bach made his discoveries, most of the people who have used the remedies have used them for self-help. Sometimes self-help means a straightforward application of a single remedy. At other times it means dealing with quite complex problems that require many different mixes of remedy. Here are some examples.

Beatrice's story

I have a long-term degenerative condition, and frequently suffer extreme exhaustion. Such was the case recently when I had a lot of planting to do in the garden. I decided to take some Olive.

After half an hour nothing seemed to be happening and so I felt that I must press on regardless. I completed the work that had to be done – it took about three hours – and suddenly I realised that I was not tired at all.

I initially expected to get a sudden surge of energy after taking the Olive. Now I realise it doesn't work like that. I got on with the work and the tiredness just wasn't there any more.

Claire's story

Recently I had to go into hospital for major surgery, and was very apprehensive, as I dread pain. From the day I knew my admission date I took Water Violet (my type remedy), with Mimulus for my specific fears.

I found this significantly reduced my apprehension, so that I faced the ordeal calmly and with happiness that it would soon be over, rather than dreading its approach. I am glad to say that I came through, feeling that my fear of pain had been unfounded. The most I suffered in that way was minor discomfort.

Joshua's story

I come from a family with numerous mental and emotional disorders. In my early teens I began having episodes of deep depression, like a dark, gloomy cloud that came out of nowhere and parked itself over my head. By the time I was 20 I decided that allopathic medicine had only drugs to offer, so I determined to find my own answers.

Homoeopathic treatment, acupuncture and herbs all helped to some degree, but despite all attempts the thread of the depression persisted.

Then I bought a set of Bach flower remedies and a book on how to use them. The description of Mustard fitted my symptoms perfectly, so I began to take it. The periods of depression lessened and became further and further apart. I continued with this remedy for nine months, at which time I stopped taking it. The depression has not returned at all.

Sheila's story

My son was born by caesarean section after a full day in labour. Although I had been greatly looking forward to having the baby, I could not shake off feelings of depression, exhaustion, fear and over-anxiety about the child. My mind was running riot with imaginary fears. I even had a few panic attacks, which I've never had before.

After two months of this a friend dosed me with a mix of Bach remedies – I can't remember what they were – and at the same time I started taking iron tablets. The mental exhaustion went, and I put my recovery down to the extra iron.

However, seven months after the birth I was still suffering from over-anxiety, irritability, feelings of not being able to get everything done and a consequent fear of losing my temper. So I got some books on the remedies – *The Twelve Healers, Questions and Answers* and *Bach Flower Remedies Step by Step* – and from these I decided that I needed Cherry Plum, Hornbeam and Mimulus.

I dosed myself day and night (the baby wakes for two or three feeds at night) and after two-and-a-half weeks I began to feel more mellow. After three weeks I felt so much myself again that I felt no need to continue with the remedies. In fact I feel better than I used to – and I have an increased sense of enjoyment of my baby, instead of an over-anxious care.

Ray's story

At the age of 21 I had a severe nervous breakdown, which left me incapable of communicating with the outside world. It meant that I could not go outside my house for nearly a year without suffering anxiety attacks.

The breakdown was brought on by pressure from my father, who was a very wealthy and successful businessman. He tried to mould my character so that I would follow in his footsteps. My personality was being suppressed and I finally cracked.

I was prescribed Valium, which is no cure but is a temporary relief. My mother then contacted a top psychiatrist who was very understanding and helpful. After two months I came off the Valium and tried to combat my fears with his help and advice alone. For ten years I slowly improved, but I had reached an emotional barrier: I could go out and meet people and do all the things needed to survive and work in this world, but I still got anxiety attacks.

I tried homoeopathy, but after a year I was still at the barrier. I became depressed as I thought I had reached the limits of my recovery. I saw the prospect of living the rest of my life with irrational and uncontrollable anxiety.

Then I discovered Bach. After three months my life had changed so dramatically that even now I can't believe it. The emotional barrier dropped and I felt free. It was fantastic – a new life.

Up until my breakdown I had been an engineer, but during the ten years that followed I discovered creativity within myself and started writing music. Now I am acting under a professional name and appeared recently on TV. You can imagine what an achievement that is for a man who once couldn't even walk out the front door.

Practitioners

From time to time people using the remedies get stuck, and when that happens they have the option to go to see a professional practitioner. This might be someone who is using the remedies as one of many therapeutic approaches, or someone who specialises entirely in Dr Bach's system. In either case the results can repay the investment, as the following examples show.

Natalie's story

At her consultation Natalie sat on the edge of her chair and looked nervous, although she smiled all the time. She told the practitioner that she was feeling tense and anxious about her forthcoming college examinations. She felt frightened of failing and letting herself down and of the effects a failure would have on her future plans. Yet at the same time she was finding it hard to get motivated enough to study, and kept discovering excuses to put off looking at her books.

As the consultation went on she seemed to be uncomfortable with having to talk about herself, although she continued to smile and laugh at every opportunity. She said she was a confident person on the whole and expected to succeed. However, she had taken on a lot recently – as well as her college work she was holding down a part-time job in a supermarket and learning to drive – and she was feeling more under pressure than usual, which perhaps accounted for her lack of confidence about the exams.

The way Natalie presented herself during the consultation, wearing a smile even as she was describing how anxious she felt, was a clear indication for Agrimony. Larch was the first choice for the lack of confidence and fear of failure, but when this remedy was explained to Natalie she made it clear that she felt she was a confident person – and it was true that she hadn't hesitated to take on a large number of commitments. When she heard the indications for Elm, however, she agreed at once that this described how she was feeling: a capable person who had taken on too much. Elm was chosen instead of Larch, and Mimulus because of her specific fears about her future if the exams did not go well.

Finally, Hornbeam was added to Natalie's mix to help her over her tendency to put off revising.

The exams went well; but the fallout in other areas of her life was in some ways more interesting. As she took the remedies over a number of weeks she found that she became more comfortable with acknowledging and expressing the way she felt. On one occasion she talked through a problem with four friends, something that she would never have done before, and on another she was able to discuss a difficult situation with her mother and find a resolution, whereas before she would have pretended that all was well. People commented on how relaxed she seemed compared with her normal self, and wondered to what they should attribute the changes.

Stephanie's story

Stephanie came for help because she was struggling with an unusually large workload, which was causing her a great deal of unhappiness and stress. As a board member of a prestigious professional organisation she had landed the job of arranging their next international convention. She was an efficient woman with a forceful personality and was used to organising other people. But she quickly found that this task took all her waking moments and brought her into conflict with other equally strong people. The job was all the more difficult because she was not getting any help or advice from the person who had been in charge before her – a fact that she resented. As the months went on she began to put on weight, and felt tired, frustrated and tense.

The main remedies that the practitioner selected for Stephanie were: Elm, for her feeling of being overwhelmed by the demands being made on her; Beech, to help her feel more tolerance for the views of other people in the organisation; Mimulus, for the specific fears that she had of things going wrong; Willow, for her resentment over having been put in this situation; Oak, because she was struggling on despite her exhaustion. White Chestnut was also given, to help overcome the obsessive, repetitive thoughts that kept her awake at night, which were contributing to her tiredness.

As Stephanie said later on, as soon as she started taking these remedies she felt things begin to change inside her. Instead of seeing her task as a looming nightmare she actually began to enjoy herself. By the time the convention came around she was a tower of strength, enthusiasm and diplomacy. Nobody who saw her in action could have guessed how negative she had felt only a few months before.

Gordon's story

Gordon was 24 years old. For the past seven years he had been taking drugs for depression, but he remained full of fear and more recently had suffered physical side effects from the treatment. His doctor advised him to try Bach remedies alongside his orthodox treatment, which is why he approached a Bach practitioner for help.

Gordon arrived at the consultation in a state of near terror. His eyes were wide open and he was sweating heavily. He explained that his depression and anxiety left him unable to travel by himself. He was too frightened to take the bus. His father had to drive him to work. His father had driven him to the consultation as well.

Gordon said that he kept his fears hidden from his co-workers. He pretended to be happy and cheerful so that they would not find out how he really felt. He was going out with a girl who was sympathetic to his plight, but he felt guilty because of the effect that his problems were having on their relationship.

The first treatment bottle mixed for Gordon contained: Rock Rose for his terror of travelling and of having an accident; Aspen for the more generalised, vague sense of foreboding; Agrimony for the way he hid his real feelings; White Chestnut because his thoughts were out of control and his mind was never still.

The next consultation took place a month later. He took the lift up to the practitioner's rooms, and said that it was the first time in three years that he had ridden in a lift. Generally the fears were less pronounced, although they still surfaced from time to time. After taking the remedies he felt more aware of the source of his fears: it was a fear of being trapped that caused the anxiety.

He mentioned again feeling guilty over the effect that his fears had on his girlfriend and also a general lack of confidence.

The fear now had a definite name. He was given Mimulus this time, and Pine was added for the guilt. The lack of confidence, which caused him to avoid challenges, indicated a need for Larch. White Chestnut was again used to calm his worrying thoughts.

Treatment with the remedies continued over the next few months. At each stage the practitioner introduced one or two new remedies to deal with newly identified aspects of his mental state. As the fear remedies did their work, so the importance of Larch grew. 'I think of all the remedies Larch was the one that helped me most,' he told his practitioner. 'I have got back my natural courage to do things, and now I feel strong and fearless.'

Eileen's story

At 68, Eileen had been taking a number of different antidepressant drugs for more than three years, most recently Prozac. Despite this she remained very tearful. She suffered from loss of appetite, insomnia and anxiety, accompanied by digestive problems and a chronic stomach ache.

At the first consultation Eileen appeared nervous and struggled to control her feelings. She described having been a shy and nervous little girl, whose childhood was full of panic, tears and stomach aches. As the youngest of 11 siblings she had ended up taking care of her eldest sister's children and had missed out on school.

Since then she had married, moved to a new country and had four children of her own, one of whom was autistic. This son lived in a residential home. Eileen was eaten up with worry over what might happen to him in the future when she would no longer be there to look out for him.

Knowing a little about Eileen's childhood made it easier to identify Mimulus as a probable type remedy for her – a selection that was backed up by her current nervousness and many incidental fears. Her extreme sense of hopelessness after taking so many drugs with no improvement indicated Sweet Chestnut. The various unresolved traumas in her past led the practitioner to include Star of Bethlehem as well. Finally, her worries over her son's welfare indicated Red Chestnut.

Eileen dropped in on the practitioner about ten days later, bringing a piece of cake as a thank you. At the next regular appointment she explained further what had happened. On her third day on the remedies her appetite had started to come back. Her stomach had not hurt once, and the pain had gone. On an emotional level she felt calmer and more alive, and was able to enjoy being with her grandchildren more.

No further remedies seemed necessary. There was no relapse, and in concert with her doctor Eileen was able to plan a reduction in her use of antidepressants.

Karen's story

Karen was referred to a Bach practitioner by a friend of hers – a client of the same practitioner. During the consultation she spoke quietly and calmly, but tears came to her eyes every so often, and she kept her head bowed.

Karen talked about her relationship with her son, aged three. She described feelings of anger and resentment. She felt it was unfair that she could no longer enjoy her old lifestyle now that she had a child. She often lost her temper with him, then felt guilty and depressed at her lack of control. Things were so bad that her son was starting to stutter, while she was more and more afraid to be left alone with him for fear of what might happen.

It was important to reassure Karen that her negative thoughts did not make her a bad person. She was taking a brave step by acknowledging the way she felt and seeking to do something about it. It was important too to suggest that she seek out extra counselling from someone qualified in the area of child abuse and family relationships, as much for her own protection as for her son's.

Karen's fears of losing control and doing harm to her son were clear indicators for Cherry Plum. The resentment and bitterness indicated Willow, and the guilt and self-reproach suggested Pine. In addition the practitioner suggested she keep a bottle of the crisis 'rescue' blend to hand, for herself and her son, to take whenever the atmosphere between them became too tense.

At the second consultation the relationship between mother and son had improved. They were enjoying each other's company again. Karen's violent, uncontrolled impulses had faded to a marked degree. At the same time she had begun to see more clearly where her feelings were coming from.

For the first time Karen was able to talk about the sexual abuse she had received from her stepfather. She was full of hatred for this man. At the same time, she tried to control other people, perhaps to compensate for the powerlessness of her early years. Holly and Vine were indicated, and added to the mix.

As the treatment progressed Cherry Plum was no longer needed. Karen no longer feared doing violence to her son or being alone with him. However, she continued to take the other remedies for some time. They helped her come to terms with her feelings about her stepfather – feelings that she explored in more depth in a series of independent sessions with a counsellor.

Using the remedies with other therapies

As some of these stories suggest, people often use the remedies to complement other treatments. We have seen that the Bach system doesn't target physical symptoms directly. It focuses on the emotional and spiritual state of the person. Because it works on a different level, the Bach system doesn't interfere with other modalities, whether orthodox or alternative.

Complementary health professionals in many different disciplines frequently offer Bach remedies as a helpful addition to their main therapy. Someone who is giving aromatherapy massages might add one or more remedies to the massage oil. Even better, she might give her client a treatment bottle to take away with her. That way her client gets the continuing benefits of regular remedy doses in between sessions on the massage table.

More and more orthodox medical practitioners – particularly people who have daily hands-on contact with patients, such as midwives, nurses and general practitioners – also see the benefits of using the remedies alongside their drug- or technology-based approaches. Patients find comfort in having something to hand that they can take as often as they need. The remedies help treat the underlying causes of stress while the physical fallout is eased using more direct intervention.

This kind of complementary use of the Bach system works well in the vast majority of cases. The remedies are non-toxic and will not react or interfere with other medicines. The only possible contraindications are to do with the fact that the concentrated stock remedies are usually preserved in alcohol. Even here, the amount of alcohol in a dose can be reduced to near zero if we dilute the remedies before use.

We will learn how to dilute remedies – and look more closely at the alcohol question – in Chapter 6. Before that, however, we will get a deeper insight into the system if we spend some time looking at a few underlying concepts. What do the remedies actually do to us? And is it possible to explain how they go about doing it? We will try to answer these questions in the next chapter.

3

How Do Bach Flower Remedies Work?

Self-help and self-improvement

Ideally, the first therapist who selects Bach remedies for you will explain what she has chosen and why. She will know that at some point you may want to use the system yourself. If you buy a book like this one and start to choose remedies without the assistance of a practitioner then you are taking the self-help route right from the start. But what does self-help with Bach remedies really mean?

Many people read 'self-help' as 'self-improvement'. We are all familiar with books and DVDs that promise a new you in 20 days or offer to advance our career, love-life and spiritual and physical development to such an extent that we won't recognise ourselves. This vision of self-help means, in effect, not being who we are. It means adopting a set of ideal characteristics that will turn us into someone else. It means copying another personality or following someone else's blueprint. Self-help becomes self-annihilation: out with the old you and in with the new.

Being yourself

Dr Bach's system is different. Instead of a new you, the promise here is to introduce you to someone you might not have met for some time: the old you. Self-help in this conception means helping yourself to be yourself.

Dr Bach believed that we are here on earth to learn from who we are. Our time on the planet is an opportunity to discover our strengths and work on our weaknesses. We can't do this by becoming someone else. Instead, the task is to find out who we really are, be that person and find the richness inherent in our lives.

The higher self and the personality

Why should we want so much to be who we are?

For Dr Bach the answer to this question lay in his belief that there was more to us than our everyday personalities. He expressed this idea by breaking down the whole of people's emotional and spiritual beings into two complementary halves.

One aspect is the higher self – this is, if you like, the spiritual aspect of our selves, our soul, the divine spark. Dr Bach believed the higher self to be immortal and perfect. Its role he defined as that of a guide, leading the whole person towards perfection.

The higher self does not manifest directly in our world. Instead it incarnates through the personality, the second of the two components that make up a whole person. The personality can be defined as our everyday mental self. It is here to help the higher self express and achieve perfection for the whole. It does this by experiencing life and overcoming difficulties, gaining wisdom along the way.

However, the personality has a limited autonomy of its own. Instead of completing its mission it can be led astray by outside influences, or fall into error under its own volition and begin to follow a path that diverges from that laid down by the higher self. The personality in this case has lost its way. It is no longer itself. It can be said to be out of balance with its own life's purpose.

The concept of unity

As well as being true to ourselves, which means being true to our higher selves, Dr Bach also believed that we need to live in right relations with other people and with the universe as a whole.

In the twenty-first century we know more than our ancestors about the interdependence of life on earth. We hardly need Dr Bach to remind us that we are bound together and that humanity forms a unified whole. Instantaneous communication means we are always in touch with each other. Twitter demonstrates every day that when we are cruel towards another person, the wrong action will, in the end, come back against us. Twenty-four-hour news is the means by which something that hurts one person in a faraway place can cause emotional pain to millions. People burning trees in Brazil change the weather in Europe.

It is less obvious, perhaps, that one way of hurting other people is to control them. Each individual has his or her own particular path to follow, said Dr Bach. If we interfere and divert somebody into a path of our choosing then we are disrupting the harmony of the whole by causing parts of that whole to misfire. It makes no difference that our motives are good and that we feel our influence and advice is helpful.

Imbalance and its results

Dr Bach said that there were therefore two faults that our personalities could commit. The first is to take a false path by not living the life that we are here to live. The second is to harm the whole by hurting or impeding the life of another. Both involve a state of imbalance. When we are ourselves and are living at peace with others, we are in balance. When we are not ourselves, or when we have given in to our weaknesses or when we are at war with others, we are out of balance.

Being out of balance means we are more likely to fall prey to sickness, which is the physical manifestation of this state. In the 1930s Dr Bach explained ill health in terms of the higher self's attempt to reign in the personality and prevent it from going further off the rails. A counsellor today might talk about stress-related illness and the need to find ourselves. Both would agree that if balance can be brought back, health can return – just as the sun shines in when the curtains are pulled back.

The snowball effect

That is the theory. Let's look at how things work in practice.

Imagine you do a job you love. You make furniture. You work by hand and use the best-quality materials because you enjoy the feel of the timber and the weight of well-made, precision tools. You work for yourself, don't answer to anyone, and make a comfortable living despite the fact that you only expect to sell 30 or so pieces a year. You have found your niche, and you are at peace with the world.

Your brother-in-law owns a factory 20 miles away, which produces cheap, mass-produced sets of dining-room furniture. He too enjoys his work; for him satisfaction comes from the hustle and bustle of making deals and running a successful business. He is proud of the fact that his furniture gives value for money. The people who buy it could never afford the chairs and tables you make.

One day your brother-in-law comes for a visit. At dinner he notices and likes the dining-room table, which you designed and made for yourself. Next day he offers you a very large salary – more than double what you currently earn – to join his firm and take personal charge of the design department.

You think it over. You don't want to do it, but you have always found it hard to say no to him. It is a lot of money. Reluctantly, you accept the offer.

At first you throw yourself into the new job, determined to make a success of it. In the back of your mind is the thought that you will be able to keep making your own furniture in your spare time. But the hours at the factory are long, as is the rush-hour commute to and from work. At the hour you get home the children are already in bed, and you barely have enough energy to slump in front of the television. The weekends are your only chance to spend time with the family. Your tools gather dust in the workroom.

Up to now you have got on well with your brother-in-law, in a distant kind of way. Now that you work for him the relationship changes. He is very pleasant, but he expects you to do as you are told and can be fairly abrasive if he thinks you are not pulling your weight. And if you are honest you are not pulling your weight. Your first few designs don't quite work and look even worse when they have been knocked together out of the fibreboard and cheap pine that the company uses for raw materials.

After a month or so you begin to suffer from headaches. You are taking out your frustrations on your wife and family. You hate yourself for doing it, but you are permanently on a short fuse and lose your temper before you have time to remember to keep it. A couple of times you smack the children – something you never did in the past. Tired all the time, you are beginning to lose confidence in yourself as a father and as a designer.

Eventually your health breaks down into a series of colds and attacks of flu. You feel sorry for yourself – it's all everyone else's fault. You begin to hate your brother-in-law for messing up your life, and you plan how you can take revenge.

This is a made-up story, but it shows how easy it is to be unbalanced by the things that happen to us in life. In the story, you were in balance when you were following your own path in life and making your furniture your way. Your brother-in-law was also in balance, doing work that he liked and making a positive contribution. The problem started when you allowed yourself to be deflected from your path.

When your brother-in-law made the job offer you could have said no. If you had taken the Centaury remedy, this would have helped you do so. The rest of the story would never have happened.

On the other hand, if you only turn to the remedies when the problem is already there, you may have forgotten all about the fact that the real cause was your failure to resist someone else's wishes. Instead you will be suffering from a collection of apparently unrelated mental states: guilt for neglecting your children or for not doing a good job; frustration; tiredness; a lack of confidence in your ability to do the job well. After a time, as we have seen, these feelings may also be covered up – in our example by self-pity and hatred.

In Bach flower remedy circles we call this the snowball effect. Untreated imbalances tend to build up layers of negative emotion. Once the snowball builds we lose sight of our path in life and of the original problem. There seem to be so many difficulties that we may be unsure where to begin.

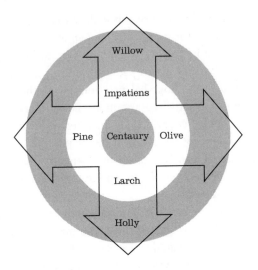

Figure 3.1 The snowball effect: how
emotional states build up in layers

Peeling the onion

How can we undo the snowball effect?

In an ideal world we wouldn't need to. We would take the one remedy we need when the first threat to our balance shows itself. A different process applies, however, if we only see the problem when the damage has been done. Bach practitioners call it peeling the onion, and it means using a series of remedy mixes to remove layers of negative emotion, one by one, so as to work back gradually to the core problem.

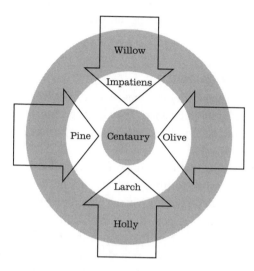

Figure 3.2 Peeling the onion: the remedies work from the outside in, until the real root of the problem is revealed

So our furniture maker might start with Holly and Willow, to resolve the bitterness and remove the desire to take revenge. That layer gone, he would be aware again of his guilt at treating the children badly and of his frustration and tiredness. Taking remedies for those states would mean that, in time, the further underlying cause would show itself – the Centaury state. The Centaury remedy would help him set his own boundaries, say no, and get back on track.

Onion peeling can be a slow method when there are many layers of emotional baggage to work through, but the process itself is valuable and worth taking time over. All sustained use of the Bach remedies is in the end a way of finding out about ourselves. Peeling the onion gives us time to learn from our mistakes so that we are less likely to repeat them in the future. We do not need to analyse ourselves to the nth degree or try to guess right away what might lie at the heart of the onion. We take the remedies we need today, and leave it to the flowers to uncover the hidden heart of the situation.

Regaining balance

As we have seen, the remedies work to peel the onion and reveal the initial imbalance. They help to restore balance so that we are once more ourselves and can resume our course in life.

This means that the action of the remedies is *restorative*, in that they work to bring us back to who we were when things began to go wrong. This in turn allows us to continue our personal path of growth and evolution.

We saw at the start of this chapter that people sometimes interpret the action of the remedies in a different way, and see them not as restorative but as *aspirational* – in other words, actually carrying out the growth and evolution for us, helping to turn us into something else.

To see how false this idea is we only have to look at what happens when we take remedies. A shy, timid person taking the correct remedy will regain a natural quiet courage that will allow him to face up to things instead of running from them. He will not turn into a flamboyant daredevil. Indeed, if a person were to take some potion to change his nature he would only be losing his balance in a different direction. Balance is not to be found at the extremes of our ups and downs. It lies at the midpoint of the seesaw, where we are who we are.

Vibrations and energy

The obvious question that arises is: how exactly do the remedies work? What is the mysterious force that restores balance to out-of-balance emotions?

There have been various theories put forward over the years. In Dr Bach's day people talked about *vibrations* and described how the vibrations of a prepared remedy echoed the natural vibrations of positive emotions. Dr Bach himself talked about vibrations at different times, although unlike some of today's theorists he did not claim to know what a vibration really was – it was just a name given to a force.

More recently the talk is of *energy* or, more often, *subtle energy* – in other words a form of energy that we have not yet succeeded in quantifying, and one that works on the spiritual and mental plane – sometimes referred to as the *subtle body*.

Dr Bach said something about theorising at the end of his research: 'They who will obtain the greatest benefit from this God-sent gift,' he wrote, 'will be those who keep it pure as it is; free from science, free from theories, for everything in nature is simple.'

The message is clear: theories about the way the remedies work don't help us use them more effectively. If anything they get in the way, because they lead to unnecessary complication of something that should be simple. However much a theory might try to incorporate fashionable scientific concepts like quantum mechanics and chaos, it will still function mostly as a metaphor. We are at liberty to pick a metaphor that seems most satisfying to us, but that doesn't mean that the metaphor we choose is truer than any other.

For the moment at least, we have to class the active property in the remedies with those other phenomena whose existence we assume every day but for which we have no truly understandable explanation. Consciousness, gravity, free will, superstrings, black holes, the nature of life and matter: science and philosophy are littered with concepts for which we can only advance metaphorical and hypothetical explanations. If the remedies appear strange and unaccountable, they are in good company.

Like beautiful music

Perhaps the best metaphor for the action of the remedies – 'best' in the sense of being the one that has the most explanatory power – is Dr Bach's own. He spoke of the remedies as being like beautiful music, or any gloriously uplifting thing that gives us inspiration. Their action, he said, is to open up our channels for reception of our spiritual self.

The analogy with music is a good one. A piece of music that means a lot to us moves us. It calls out to something that is in us already. We feel differently from the way we felt before. We are not changed from who we were, but a different side of us responds and gains energy.

This is exactly what happens when we take the remedies. They don't put qualities into us that were not there before. Instead they encourage the positive emotions that were already in us, so that they become strong enough to overwhelm and drive out the negative feelings that were dragging us out of balance.

The music metaphor is so good that it can explain other aspects of remedy use that may appear at first to be counterintuitive.

For example, many people coming to the remedies for the first time are confused by the dosage instructions (see Chapter 6). They cannot see how taking two drops of pure remedy straight from a stock bottle can possibly be the same as putting the same two drops into 30 ml of water and then taking only four drops of that extremely dilute mixture. If the remedies worked like orthodox drugs (the line marked 1 in Figure 3.3), the stronger mix would have a stronger effect. If they worked like homoeopathy (marked 2), the more dilute dose would be stronger. Yet with the remedies both doses are the same. How can this be?

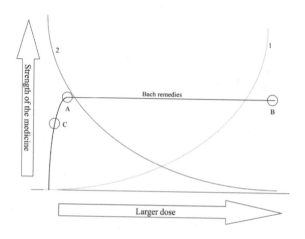

Figure 3.3 A melody is a melody: the effect of different strength doses

The answer falls into place when we think of the remedies as music. A melody remains the same whether it comes from someone playing a flute three streets away, or from a symphony orchestra right in the room with you. If we can hear the melody, we can hear it. The volume is irrelevant.

So if we are getting the minimum dose of a remedy – four drops from a treatment bottle, marked A in Figure 3.3 – we might say that the message in the remedy is just within earshot. We don't recognise the meaning any better if we take drops straight from the stock bottle, or even drink down a whole stock bottle (B) – the broadcast may be louder but it is the same message. If we take less than the minimum dose – say two drops from the treatment bottle instead of four (C) – those of us who are less sensitive may no longer hear the message with so much certainty: the remedies work less effectively, or not at all.

The same analogy helps us understand what is happening when we mix remedies together. Selecting and blending together the remedies we need is like combining different melody lines into a single musical arrangement.

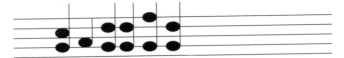

Figure 3.4 A harmonious selection of remedies

If we select aright, the main tune comes through very strongly and is easy to hear. If we put in a couple of remedies that we don't need, the sound of those remedies makes it harder to hear the notes produced by the others. And if we mix too many remedies together – more than the recommended six or seven – we could have real trouble picking out any melody at all.

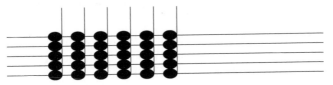

Figure 3.5 Too many remedies

In Dr Bach's day someone suggested that he might combine all his remedies to produce a single elixir for everyone. He tried, and found that the resultant mix didn't work. In the same way, playing all the notes available all at the same time produces white noise. No music can be heard at all.

Are Bach remedies placebos?

As they do with most forms of complementary medicine, sceptics sometimes accuse the remedies of being nothing but placebos, which only work because the person taking them believes in them. The same results would be achieved, they say, if there were no flowers used at all.

There is a measure of truth in this. All medicines and therapies, including the strongest of orthodox drugs, benefit from the placebo effect. If we think something is good for us we tend to feel better when we take it. When we have a headache and take an aspirin, part of the effect of the aspirin is to build up our confidence that the headache will go.

The strength of the placebo effect can be demonstrated by looking at its opposite – the nocebo effect. The nocebo effect is the power of negative thinking. We can demonstrate it by giving a drug that we know to be effective to people who believe that the drug doesn't work. Alternatively we can tell them that we are giving them a dummy drug. If people with a headache take an aspirin believing it to be nothing but a sugar pill, the nocebo effect means they are less likely to feel any relief.

The nocebo effect could explain why people who believe in witchcraft and black magic are at risk from sorcerers. Their belief in the power of spells is such that they really do fall ill and die if someone lays a curse on them. Similarly, sceptics who take a Bach flower remedy while firmly convinced that they do not work are more likely than others to have their prejudices confirmed. They are no different from people who don't believe in the power of aspirin or antibiotics.

There is, of course, more to orthodox medicine than belief and the same is true of the remedies. We know this because both approaches work on many people who don't believe in them. Sceptics have been helped by flower remedies despite themselves, and people who have been given the remedies without their knowledge have also benefitted. (It may not be morally defensible to treat someone without consent, but it isn't unknown between husband and wife.)

Furthermore, the remedies have been shown to be effective with animals, plants and very young babies; we will see this in Chapter 7. It can't easily be demonstrated that animals and babies respond to suggestion, especially in cases where they are not aware that they are being treated with anything. The obvious hypothesis must be that the remedies are potent in their own right, over and above the placebo effect that they share with medicine in general.

4

The Remedies

Now that we know something about the background to this system of medicine, we can look in more detail at the individual remedies. There are 38 in all, plus the so-called 'thirty-ninth' remedy, with which we start.

The emergency formula

The best-known remedy in the system is a formula put together by Dr Bach. Sold under different trade names, including Rescue Remedy, Five Flower Remedy and Recovery Remedy, it is a mix of five essences:

1. Star of Bethlehem for shock

2. Rock Rose for terror

3. Clematis for faint, far-away, disconnected feelings

4. Impatiens for agitation

5. Cherry Plum for loss of self-control.

This combination is unique in Dr Bach's system. He taught his colleagues not to use ready-mixed formulas and to look instead at the personality and emotional state of each individual to select a personal blend. Nevertheless, he was aware that there would be emergencies when something would be needed at once and there would not be time to select specific remedies. He created the emergency formula with occasions like these in mind.

Dr Bach used the formula on several occasions and always carried a bottle in his pocket. Once, when he was living in Cromer, a lifeboat rescued a man who had been strapped to a mast for five hours during a storm. Many thought the sailor would die when he was finally brought to shore; he was in a delirium and stiff with cold. Dr Bach moistened his lips with the formula all the way up the beach. By the time they reached the first house the sailor was able to sit up and talk to his rescuers.

As well as being useful in this kind of crisis, the formula is also used to help overcome less dramatic situations. It can calm last-minute nerves before an exam, for example, or we can take it when we receive bad news or when we feel upset after an argument.

Linda's story

I went into labour after being induced with Pitocin, a drug that is known to make labour particularly intense and painful. After only a little progress I felt overwhelmed with the pain and felt I could not take any more. I was very scared and asked for pain relief.

My labour assistant, knowing I wanted to get by without, suggested I use Rescue Remedy. I took a dose and by the very next contraction I had calmed down, focused on the job and taken control. The pain didn't go away but I was able to manage it so that it didn't overwhelm me any more.

I took three or four more doses over the next five hours and gave birth to my son completely without pain relief and completely in control of the birth. I am sure that the remedy helped me get over my initial anxiety and have a wonderful, natural birth experience. I recommend it to all my pregnant friends.

Going beyond the emergency mix

Some remedy users treat Dr Bach's emergency formula as a quick fix, a kind of crutch that helps keep them functioning day to day, even when their lives are out of balance. A better approach is to think of it as a gateway to the 38 individual remedies. Using the emergency formula on a daily basis won't do any harm, but it won't deal with underlying problems. If we find we need rescuing on a regular basis, it's a good idea to think about why that might be.

For example, we might ease unexpected exam nerves with Rescue Remedy or Five Flower Remedy. But suppose our problem is caused by a chronic lack of confidence, or we are nervous because we have once again failed to revise properly. A pre-mixed emergency combination is unlikely to do much good. A good practitioner would want to select a personal mix to address the root of the problem.

The seven groups

In his last book, *The Twelve Healers and Other Remedies*, Dr Bach sorted the 38 remedies into seven groups, as remedies for:

1. fear

2. uncertainty

3. insufficient interest in present circumstances

4. loneliness

5. oversensitivity to influences and ideas

6. despondency or despair

7. over-care for the welfare of others.

We don't need to learn which remedy is in which group, because we don't need to refer to the groups when making a selection. We simply pick the remedies we need. Nevertheless, the groups can help us understand some of the subtler differences between remedies, so we will come back to them again at the end of this chapter.

First we will look at the 38 remedies.

Remedies for fear

There are five 'fear' remedies:

1. to treat fear of known things, things that we can name – Mimulus

2. to treat terror – Rock Rose

3. to treat fear where the cause is not known – Aspen

4. to treat the fear of losing our reason – Cherry Plum

5. to treat the fear that something will happen to a loved one – Red Chestnut.

Mimulus

The plant used to make the Mimulus remedy is *Mimulus guttatus*, the monkey flower. Mimulus grows in wet land, often at the edge of streams, and is remarkable for its large yellow flowers.

Mimulus is the remedy for everyday fears and anxieties, such as a fear of losing a job or of speaking in public, or a fear of the dark. In general, the Mimulus fear is any fear where we can name the thing that we are afraid of.

Mimulus is also associated with those types of people who tend to be nervous and shy, and who blush easily or stammer.

The remedy is taken to encourage the quiet reserves of strength and courage that lie underneath such everyday fears, so that anxieties can be faced and learnt from and overcome.

Rock Rose

The *Helianthemum nummularium* flower used to make Rock Rose is small, paper thin and a translucent pale yellow. The plant grows close to the ground, often in stony or chalky soil.

As a remedy, Rock Rose is associated with terror. The Rock Rose state is one of paralysis or panic: the thing happening is so frightening that the person is incapable of dealing with it.

The aim in taking this remedy is to reawaken the will so that we can face terror and deal with whatever is causing it. Dr Bach referred to Rock Rose as 'the rescue remedy', so it is no surprise that it was one of the first remedies he selected for his emergency mix.

Aspen

Catkins from the Aspen tree – *Populus tremula* – are the essential ingredient of the Aspen remedy. The remedy counteracts those vague, free-floating anxieties that seem to come for no reason. Aspen feelings range from a mild sense of foreboding where something seems wrong – we can't quite say what – all the way up to stark terror.

We can contrast the Aspen state with the Mimulus and Rock Rose fears – both of which have causes that can be named.

The remedy works to strengthen our ability to trust life and ourselves, so that we come to realise how faith can overcome any fear.

Cherry Plum

Cherry Plum comes from the spring blossoms of the tree *Prunus cerasifera*. The flowers are as white as snow and as numerous as snowflakes, and all the more welcome for being among the first to appear just as winter is ending.

The Cherry Plum remedy alleviates a very particular kind of fear, the fear of loss of reason and self-control. The person in this state may be afraid that she is about to go crazy and perhaps injure herself or someone else.

A good examples of this state is seen in toddlers having a temper tantrum. Underneath their rage lies a great fear caused by the intensity of their emotions and their inability to control them.

The action of Cherry Plum is to give us courage to confront our feelings and their causes. The emotional crisis becomes an opportunity for learning and moving on.

Red Chestnut

Red Chestnut is another remedy for a specific kind of fear, in this case an altruistic fear felt over the well-being and safety of someone else. In this state we imagine all kinds of accidents and illnesses happening, especially to people who are close to us.

Red Chestnut anxiety can become exaggerated and turn into a burden, not only to the worrier but also to the person being worried about.

The remedy is made from the pink-red flowers of *Aesculus carnea*. In the positive Red Chestnut state our confidence in the security of the people we love feeds their self-confidence and gives them renewed faith in their abilities.

Remedies for uncertainty

There are six 'uncertainty' remedies:

1. for doubting our own decisions – Cerato

2. for not being able to take decisions – Scleranthus

3. for feeling discouraged – Gentian

4. for pessimism and for giving up – Gorse

5. for when we feel tired at the thought of the things we have to do – Hornbeam

6. for uncertainty about our true path in life – Wild Oat.

Cerato

Cerato is an oddity among the 38 remedies, being the only non-naturalised plant chosen by Dr Bach. *Ceratostigma willmottianum* came originally from the Himalayas, and in the UK it only grows in gardens. At The Bach Centre, we cover the bushes up each winter to protect them from the frost – something we don't have to do for any other remedy plant. The flowers appear in the summer and are an intense blue.

The remedy made from this plant is for people who lack faith in their judgement. In the Cerato state we make decisions but, having made them, immediately doubt whether we are doing the right thing. This leads us to ask other people for advice instead of trusting our own intuition.

Cerato helps remove the doubt so that we can act in the way we feel is right for us.

Scleranthus

Scleranthus annuus is a tiny plant with green flowers. The combination of its size and colour makes it difficult to find in the wild because it blends so well with its background.

The Scleranthus remedy is for people who struggle to choose an option from the alternatives in front of them. The decision in question could be something important, such as whether to accept a new job or not, or something relatively unimportant, such as whether to wear this jacket or that –

but in all cases the Scleranthus person dithers, first choosing one option and then the other. Unlike people in the Cerato state, Scleranthus people tend not to ask for advice.

Scleranthus encourages our innate decisiveness, so that we can cut through the uncertainty and make our choice calmly and precisely.

Gentian

Gentiana amarella, the autumn gentian, is the plant used to make the Gentian remedy. The flower is a deep blue-purple, and grows in clusters on upright stems.

We take Gentian when we have suffered a setback of some kind – failing an exam, for example, or suffering an illness – and as a result feel discouraged and inclined to give up.

The effect of this remedy is to give encouragement so that we can quickly get over the setback and get on with our lives.

Gorse

Gorse is made from the intense yellow flowers of *Ulex europaeus*, which is very common on heaths and exposed hillsides.

We can think of the Gorse state as being a few steps on from Gentian. The Gentian person feels like giving up when life becomes difficult, but usually keeps going. The Gorse person makes up his mind and gives up. In a Gorse state we adopt a pessimistic, hopeless attitude, even when other people suggest possible ways out of our situation.

Taking Gorse renews hope. It encourages our natural optimism, and gives us back the faith to try again.

Hornbeam

Hornbeam is made from the flowers of the tree *Carpinus betulus*. We take it when we feel weary at the thought of starting work on something. In consequence, Hornbeam is sometimes referred to as the 'Monday morning' remedy.

Hornbeam is a remedy for procrastination, useful when we find ourselves wasting precious time that should be spent on a more important or urgent task. It strengthens our determination to take the first step, at which point the feeling of weariness tends to melt away by itself.

Note that a different remedy is required if we feel weary as a result of *having done* work. See the entry for Olive later in this chapter.

Wild Oat

Despite its name, the Wild Oat remedy is not made from an oat at all, but from a wild grass called *Bromus ramosus*.

We take Wild Oat when we feel dissatisfied and frustrated due to an inability to find our true path in life. People in a Wild Oat state have often explored many different directions, but nothing satisfies them. They know they want to do something worthwhile, so they don't lack ambition, but they are unable to say exactly what that something should be.

The Wild Oat remedy helps us listen to our inner voice and take guidance from it. Deep inside, believed Dr Bach, we know what we are here to do. Wild Oat can help us identify that true path so we can move ahead without delay.

Remedies for insufficient interest in present circumstances

There are seven remedies for people who show insufficient interest in present circumstances':

1. to restore those who live more in dreams than in reality – Clematis

2. to restore those who live in the past – Honeysuckle

3. to encourage vitality in those who are resigned to their lives – Wild Rose

4. to restore strength to those exhausted in mind and body – Olive

5. to quiet distracting, repetitive thoughts – White Chestnut

6. to lift sudden gloom that descends from a blue sky – Mustard

7. to bring to mind the lessons of experience – Chestnut Bud.

Clematis

The remedy Clematis is made from the cream-coloured flowers of the climber *Clematis vitalba*. Common names for it include old man's beard and traveller's joy.

Clematis helps to ground people who are not paying sufficient attention to the present because they are living in daydreams – either of an imaginary alternative reality or of how things will be in some vague future.

True Clematis types create magnificent plans in their heads that they never carry out in the real world. Their minds are so little anchored to reality that they sometimes fall asleep at odd moments during the day.

Taking this remedy connects us with our inner drive and sense of purpose. Anchored more in the present, we can put our plans into effect and find more interest in life's continuous present.

Honeysuckle

The plant used for this remedy is the wild pink honeysuckle, *Lonicera caprifolium.*

We can usefully compare Honeysuckle with Clematis. Both remedy states involve a drift away from the present, but while the Clematis person is lost in daydreams of the future, the Honeysuckle person is lost, or living, in the past.

People in the Honeysuckle state may be nostalgic and miss out on chances to be happy today because they are wrapped up in thoughts about yesterday. Other times they feel regret and relive painful episodes when they might have made other choices.

The Honeysuckie remedy, again like Clematis, makes it easier for us to focus our thoughts and energies on the present. We remember the pleasures and lessons of the past, but only to the extent that they contribute to the richness of life as it is.

Wild Rose

The dog rose, *Rosa canina,* is a familiar sight in many hedgerows around Britain, and is the plant Dr Bach chose for the Wild Rose remedy.

Wild Rose is a remedy for apathy and resignation. In this state we accept whatever life throws at us. We don't struggle or try to make things better. If Wild Rose came with a gesture, it would be a shrug of the shoulders.

True Wild Rose types drift through life. They tend not to feel extremes of happiness or unhappiness and just get on with whatever they have ended up doing. At times they feel that life is passing them by and it is then that the Wild Rose remedy is indicated.

Wild Rose arouses the dormant sense of vitality, enthusiasm and joy that lies somewhere within the most lackadaisical-seeming people.

Olive

Along with Vine, Olive is one of two remedies that are not prepared in the UK. It is made from the tiny white-green flowers of *Olea europaea*, which grows in many parts of Mediterranean Europe.

Olive is one of the most commonly used remedies. It helps restore our spiritual and emotional reserves when they have been exhausted by an effort of some kind. The effort concerned can be physical or mental. Exercise, hard work, illness and study can all lead to an Olive state.

Olive should not be confused with a straightforward pick me up – it won't necessarily provide a burst of energy in the way a strong coffee would. If rest and sleep is what we need, that is what it helps us towards.

White Chestnut

White Chestnut is another widely used remedy. It is made from the white flowers of *Aesculus hippocastanum*, the horse chestnut tree.

White Chestnut is associated with worrying thoughts, but 'worry' here is not a synonym of 'anxiety' and White Chestnut is not a fear remedy. The worrying thoughts of White Chestnut are thoughts that nag, beset, plague and bedevil. They stop us concentrating and thinking constructively. They recur despite our best efforts to control them and they don't lead to a conclusion. Once the chain of a White Chestnut thought has finished it starts again from the beginning.

The action of the White Chestnut remedy is to calm the mind and put us back in control of our thoughts. This allows constructive thinking. If there is a problem that needs to be addressed we are better able to find a coherent solution.

Mustard

The wild flower *Sinapis arvensis* produces the Mustard remedy, which treats the kind of down-in-the-dumps feeling that comes from nowhere and for no reason. People suffering from this state may feel that life is full of good things for them and that they should be happy, but they aren't, and they can't say why.

The remedy works to reinforce our inner sense of joy and purposefulness so that the negative clouds can disperse as quickly as they came.

Chestnut Bud

Chestnut Bud is made from the horse chestnut tree, *Aesculus hippocastanum*, which also provides the White Chestnut remedy. But while White Chestnut uses the flowers, Chestnut Bud is made early in the spring from the sticky buds, just as they are starting to open.

We take this remedy when we feel that we are not learning from our own or other people's experiences and we are repeating mistakes. A friend may be more likely to spot this tendency in us than we are ourselves, since the Chestnut Bud state is associated with unconsciousness and lack of insight.

Chestnut Bud can be seen in the person who ends a painful relationship with a violent partner, only to start a new relationship with somebody who has a similar history of violence. The lesson of life has not been learned and has to be repeated.

Chestnut Bud helps us see the patterns in our lives more clearly, so that we are less likely to reproduce any errors we made. By watching and learning from others we may be able to avoid making a mistake in the first place.

Remedies for loneliness

The 'loneliness' group is the smallest of the seven – there are three remedies under this heading:

1. to break down the walls that can build up around self-sufficient, independent people – Water Violet

2. to bring patience to the impatient – Impatiens

3. to help talkative people who are unhappy when they have to be alone – Heather.

Water Violet

The plant used to make this remedy, *Hottonia palustris*, actually belongs to the primrose family. 'Violet' only refers to the colour of the five petals on the small, delicate flowers.

Water Violet is a remedy for people who like their own company and enjoy being self-sufficient and removed from the hustle and bustle of communal life. Their neighbours may think them arrogant or snobbish and this plus their natural reclusiveness can leave them isolated and lonely.

The remedy frees up the great talents of people of this type, so that they can relate better to their fellow creatures and put their wisdom at the service of others.

Impatiens

Only the pale mauve flowers of *Impatiens glandulifera* are used to make the Impatiens remedy. Dr Bach found that the darker flowers produced by some plants don't have the same properties.

As a mood remedy Impatiens is taken to relieve impatience and agitation. The true Impatiens type is someone who keeps others away so that she can get on with her tasks faster. She is capable, intelligent and quick-witted, but in a negative state lacks the wisdom to see value in the more methodical talents of others.

The remedy acts to reinforce our hidden depths of patience and understanding. It helps us appreciate the immense potential contribution of those who live more slowly.

Heather

The Heather remedy is made from *Calluna vulgaris*, the mauve heather that grows across open moorland.

Heather helps people who have become wrapped up in their own affairs to the exclusion of everything else. They feel an overwhelming desire to talk about every detail of their lives and for this they need an audience. Dr Bach referred to Heather people as 'buttonholers' because while they talked they would literally catch hold of people by their lapels to stop them leaving.

Heather people fear loneliness. Unfortunately their incessant talking leads others to start avoiding them, so their behaviour brings about the very circumstance they fear.

Heather raises the mind above its own everyday concerns. More interest can be taken in other people's lives, so that from being a great talker the Heather person can become a wise listener.

Remedies for oversensitivity to influences and ideas

There are four 'over-sensitivity' remedies:

1. for pretending to be happy when underneath you are suffering – Agrimony

2. for doing what other people want you to do and not being able to refuse – Centaury

3. for protection against outside influences and the effects of change – Walnut

4. for feelings of suspicion, revenge and hatred – Holly.

Agrimony

Agrimony, or *Agrimonia eupatoria*, is a long spiky plant covered in tiny yellow flowers. The Agrimony remedy is aimed at people who dislike conflict and who prefer to conceal problems under a mask of good humour and cheerfulness. Agrimony people appear happy even when they are suffering inside. They will try to raise a smile out of the most painful tragedy. Sometimes they turn to drink or drugs to help keep the mask in place and seek out company in order to forget themselves.

People in this state appear brave, but their good humour is a way of not facing up to the darker side of life. The remedy helps us use humour to resolve difficult situations, rather than using it to avoid them.

Centaury

Centaurium umbellatum is an upright plant with many small, star-shaped pink flowers. These are collected to make the Centaury remedy, which is associated with people who have difficulty saying no to others.

Common examples of Centaury states include the man who follows his father's choice of career rather than his own, and the woman who entirely gives up her own life to care for an ailing relative.

Taking this remedy doesn't make us callous or uncaring. It simply allows us the freedom and strength to draw boundaries and live our own lives. The positive Centaury state is one of freedom from the unreasonable demands of others.

Walnut

The smaller female flowers of *Juglans regia* go to make up the Walnut remedy; the larger male catkins are not used.

The remedy has two related uses. First, we might take it to help us adjust to changes, when unsettled by a move to a new job or a new neighbourhood, for example. It is equally useful during natural periods of transition such as teething and weaning and the menopause. In relation to this kind of use Walnut is called 'the link-breaker', because it eases the transition from one stage of life to another.

The second use is to give protection against outside influences that could lead us astray. If we decide to take a new job and live abroad, for example, the negative opinions of friends and relations might hold us back. This would be a time to take Walnut.

The action of the remedy is to strengthen our self-belief and confidence. We are able to move ahead without being unduly affected by the thoughts, beliefs and circumstances that surround us.

Holly

Much less well known than the famous red berries that develop from them, the tiny white flowers of *Ilex aquifolium* play the starring role in the Holly remedy.

We select Holly when we feel suspicious of other people and develop negative feeling towards them, such as hatred, envy and the desire to take revenge for actual or imagined wrongs. Holly is the remedy of love: it strengthens our understanding of others and helps us to be open and generous, even to people who really are acting wrongly towards us.

Many people also think of Holly as the remedy for anger, but this is only partly true. Holly certainly helps where anger is based on a strong and sustained desire to hurt somebody. But anger comes in many flavours – Willow, Cherry Plum and Impatiens are some alternatives – and we need to identify the cause and style of somebody's anger before we can choose the right remedy. For example, we would normally select Vervain for a righteous, altruistic anger based on a feeling that there has been an injustice.

Remedies for despondency or despair

The 'despondency or despair' group is the largest of Dr Bach's seven categories; it contains eight remedies:

1. to give us the confidence to try, and not fear failure – Larch

2. to help us be responsible for our actions without destroying ourselves with guilt – Pine

3. to restore confidence when our responsibilities weigh heavily on us – Elm

4. to give hope in the darkest moments – Sweet Chestnut

5. to overcome shock and loss – Star of Bethlehem

6. to lift us out of self-pity and towards generosity – Willow

7. to give us the strength to go on and the wisdom to rest – Oak

8. to help us when we feel we need cleansing – Crab Apple.

Larch

The Larch remedy comes from the catkins of *Larix decidua*. The tree is unusual in that it is the only conifer that sheds its leaves in autumn.

Larch increases the confidence levels of people who are convinced they will fail. True Larch types feel that they are not as talented or capable as other people. They sometimes use this feeling as an excuse for never trying to succeed.

The action of the remedy is to remove the fear of failure, so that the person can get more from life and not be worried by the eventual outcome.

Pine

The tree used to make the Pine remedy is the Scots Pine, *Pinus sylvestris* – a common sight in woodlands.

Pine is the remedy for guilt. When we are in a Pine state we tend to blame ourselves for everything that goes wrong. We may even feel guilty when in fact someone else was at fault.

Pine replaces the destructiveness of guilt with a more positive sense of responsibility and fairness. Where something really is our fault we are able to accept the blame in a more constructive way. Where the fault lies elsewhere, we no longer feel obliged to carry the burden for other people.

Elm

Since Dutch elm disease arrived in the UK the common elm tree *Ulmus procera* is no longer so common. Fortunately a few colonies survive, and younger trees often flower for a time before they eventually succumb to the disease.

As a remedy, Elm helps during those crises of confidence that come when we take on too many duties. The Elm state is one in which we doubt our ability to cope with all the demands being made on us.

We can usefully contrast Elm with Larch, which we introduced earlier in this section. Both are confidence remedies, but Larch people tend to avoid responsibility because they have no faith in their ability. This is a state of mind very different to that of the Elm person, who starts out confident of success. Indeed, their faith in themselves is the very thing that leads them to take on too much.

The remedy works to restore our faith in our ability. The Elm state is usually a temporary one in any case. Taking the remedy speeds it on its way all the faster.

Sweet Chestnut

This remedy is made from the long yellow catkins of *Castanea sativa*, the chestnut tree. It is aimed at people who have reached the end of the road and can no longer see any way out of their predicament. The Sweet Chestnut state is extreme and once seen there is no doubt of it. It is utter anguish, a total despair that comes when nothing offers an escape.

There are no easy answers or quick fixes for someone in this state. What the remedy can do, however, is bring a ray of light into the darkness. This alone can be enough to bring comfort.

Star of Bethlehem

The white flower of *Ornithogalum umbellatum* provides the remedy for shock and the after-effects of shock. Star of Bethlehem helps to soothe the trauma associated with hearing bad news, or witnessing or being involved in accidents. It also helps people who feel the pang of a great loss, including the death of a loved one.

These indications explain why this remedy is an important ingredient in Dr Bach's emergency formula. As a single remedy, however, Star of Bethlehem can help us come to terms with traumas that happened many years before, even in early childhood; it isn't just for immediate emergency use.

Star of Bethlehem consoles and comforts, even in moments of great distress.

Willow

There are many varieties of willow tree in England and Wales. The one Dr Bach chose for the Willow remedy was *Salix vitellina*, the golden osier, so called because in winter the leafless twigs turn bright yellow.

Willow helps when we feel sorry for ourselves and blame our misfortunes on other people. Perhaps we are resentful, feeling that life is not fair to us in particular, or we may begrudge others their success and happiness.

Willow lifts us out of this negative state so that we feel more generous about what other people do right and more aware of the things that we ourselves do wrong.

Left alone the negative Willow state tends to be self-perpetuating, as self-pity and resentment feed off each other. With the help of the remedy we can break the cycle and see things in a truer light.

Oak

The Oak remedy is made using the tiny scarlet-tipped female flowers of *Quercus robur*, the common oak. The much larger male flowers are not used.

Like the tree, which stands four-square in the countryside and supports more species than any other in England, Oak people are reliable, strong, slow and steady. They have the ability to take on immense responsibility and can work long into the night without ever stopping or increasing their pace.

Their immense strength is, however, the key to their downfall. Oaks never know when they are beaten. They struggle on long after they should rest. Oak people never bend, but they can break.

The remedy works in two related ways. On the one hand, it helps recharge our energies when we have exhausted ourselves with unceasing effort. On the other, it helps us measure our lives and efforts more sensibly, so that we can profit from what has happened. We learn to make space to rest. We learn that it's OK to rely on others from time to time.

Crab Apple

This remedy comes from *Malus pumila*, a crab apple tree often found in hedgerows. The flowers are a delicate light pink inside and darker outside and grow in clusters of half a dozen or so.

Crab Apple is known as the cleansing remedy. It is useful when we feel there is something unclean or unpleasant about our bodies or ourselves. Feeling contaminated by a sickness is one possible Crab Apple state, or we might feel dirtied by an unpleasant sexual experience, or say we don't like something about the way we look.

Crab Apple also helps with contaminating thoughts and obsessive behaviours. Continual hand-washing is the obvious example, but Crab Apple can be used to help any mental state where we over-concentrate on one or two details at the expense of more important concerns. A candidate for Crab Apple could be the man who straightens the pictures hanging in his house every day, yet hardly notices that the walls are about to collapse.

The remedy helps us accept ourselves. We become aware that there is clarity and light in all of us. We attend more to things of lasting value and less to appearance.

Remedies for over-care for the welfare of others

There are five 'over-care' remedies:

1. when we want to be close to our loved ones, and find it hard to let go – Chicory

2. when we are filled with enthusiasm and want to convert other people to our way of life – Vervain

3. when we force other people to do things our way – Vine

4. when everyone else is stupid and wrong – Beech

5. when we strive for personal perfection and to set an example – Rock Water.

Chicory

The Chicory remedy is made from the beautiful blue-violet flowers of *Chicorium intybus*.

As Chicory people we want to stay close to the family and friends whom we love. In order to remain the centre of their lives we offer insistent, unwanted help and advice or interfere and act hurt and upset if we don't get all the attention we feel we deserve. Chicory people can be manipulative and sometimes resort to emotional blackmail.

The Chicory state is all about love, in its way, but it's a distorted love in which our own feelings become too important. Taking the remedy allows love to flow outwards, as it should. We can give without thought of reward and usually feel happier – and more loved – as a result.

Vervain

Verbena officinalis is an upright plant with scattered clusters of tiny pale mauve flowers. These are used to make the Vervain remedy.

The key to Vervain is over-enthusiasm. True Vervain types are perfectionists who throw themselves, body and soul, into any task they undertake. They are often full of energy but risk exhaustion due to their inability to switch off.

Vervain types like to persuade and change people's minds. They tend to be committed to campaigns built around issues of principle and social justice, and they enjoy a good argument. When out of balance, though, they begin to lose the ability to hear the other side. Their enthusiasm shades into fanaticism.

Taking the remedy restores balance and flexibility of mind. We learn to maintain our enthusiasms in an open-hearted way, and how to switch off and rest.

Vine

Like Olive, which we met earlier, the Vine remedy is prepared in southern Europe, where it grows wild, and not in the UK. *Vitis vinifera's* flowers look like miniature clusters of tiny green grapes, and grapes are what they will become if left unpicked into the late summer.

Vine helps people who sometimes use their talents and force of character to dominate others. Instead of trying to convince through argument, a negative Vine will not really care what other people think as long as they do what they are told.

The action of the remedy is to encourage the positive side of leadership. Instead of being a tyrant, the Vine person grows into a guide – someone who is willing to encourage the freedom of others.

Beech

The beech tree *Fagus sylvatica* is a common sight in English woods, and its flowers – male and female – give us the Beech remedy.

We can take Beech when we find it difficult to sympathise with other people and the way they live. In a Beech state we are sure of the rightness of what we do and don't understand why anyone would want to live differently. We indulge in criticism, condemning what we don't understand instead of trying to see life through other eyes.

The remedy won't affect our sense of right and wrong or lower our high ideals. But it does help us see the good within other people so that we can tolerate differences more easily. Back in balance, we are less tense and less irritable.

Rock Water

Rock Water is an oddity among the 38 flower remedies, because it is not made using a flower. Instead it is the water from an unspoilt healing spring, prepared using the sun method.

We benefit from this remedy when we try too hard to be perfect. In a Rock Water state we set ourselves so many rules and targets that we end up stripping pleasure out of life. In part we do this because we hope others might notice our example and be inspired to follow it.

When very out of balance we become martyrs to our beliefs and take a perverse pleasure in living a life devoid of joy.

As with Beech, this remedy is not about lowering our standards. What it does is to bring us back into touch with our essential humanity. None of us can be gods here on earth. The remedy teaches the humility needed to be human and less than perfect.

Using the groups

The seven groups can be used to work out differences between apparently similar remedies. Here are a couple of examples.

Example one: Gorse and Sweet Chestnut

Key words for Gorse often include 'hopelessness' and 'despair'. Sweet Chestnut is also a remedy for people who have no hope and Dr Bach put it into the 'despondency or despair' group. So far, so similar. We might expect Gorse to be in the same category, but instead Dr Bach listed it under 'uncertainty'.

How is Gorse a type of uncertainty? The answer must be that people in a Gorse state lack a sense of conviction. They don't believe that they can get better, do better or find a way out of their predicament. Their problem is a lack of faith. If they could regain their faith – their sense of certainty – they would in fact be able to move on.

Sweet Chestnut, on the other hand, is for people who are genuinely in despair and without hope. They haven't decided to give up due to a lack of faith, as the Gorse person has, but have been forced into a corner where there is no way out. That is why this remedy, and not Gorse, appears in the 'despondency or despair' group.

Example two: Beech and Impatiens

Both remedies are given to irritable people. We find Beech listed under 'over-care for the welfare of others'. So in a Beech state we genuinely care that other people are not doing things the right way. Because we care we take the trouble to point out where they are going wrong – we criticise and condemn because their behaviour bothers us.

Impatiens on the other hand is a 'loneliness' remedy. In an Impatiens state our focus is on ourselves. Instead of criticising a mistake – and in the process explaining where somebody went wrong – we are more likely to take a job over and do it ourselves so as to have it done quicker. We will not take the time to criticise, because we don't care if other people do the wrong thing – as long as it only affects them.

The origins of the cream

In the early 1960s, Nora Weeks mixed Dr Bach's emergency formula of five remedies into a cream, along with Crab Apple, and made it available commercially. The cream was widely used on bruises, cuts and skin problems of various kinds and remains a quick and convenient way of applying the crisis mix externally.

At first sight the cream looks like a violation of the principle that the Bach remedies treat emotional states and not physical conditions. What is the theory behind it?

When Dr Bach was alive he sometimes applied the remedies to burns, bruises and wounds. In addition to giving a mix by mouth – Vervain if there was over-enthusiasm, perhaps, or Olive or Gentian if there was tiredness or discouragement – the patient might be given extra drops via a cold compress or lotion. In the very early stages of his practice Dr Bach occasionally selected different remedies for external and internal use. Later, when he was sure the emotional state was the most reliable guide, he would use same mix.

External use of personal mixes still happens today, although the remedies are enough when taken internally and most people rely on that method alone. Still, when we have an accident of some kind the first thing we reach for is the crisis formula. Many of us, in addition to swallowing the drops, find it helpful to drip them onto wasp stings and minor burns. Just as the crisis formula is the most ingested of the remedies, so it is the one that is most often used externally.

At the simplest level, then, Nora Weeks put the cream together as a convenience, a way of making it easier to apply the crisis formula, in an emergency, to the skin. She added Crab Apple because it helps people who feel there is something wrong with their appearance. It had to be a useful extra in a preparation that would be used on bruises, bites and bumps.

Like the crisis formula drops, the cream is neither a replacement for a personal mix of remedies nor a solution to a specific emotional state. Still less is it a cure for eczema or any other medical condition. Having said this, wonderful results have been achieved that show just how closely emotional and physical health are linked.

Hesta's story

Due to an accident my foot has had an open wound for 18 years. I've had several skin grafts, five in total, but none totally successful.

I bought and tried the cream and in a matter of days I saw a difference. Now, seven weeks on, my foot is healed – no more bleeding or worry in case of infection. It's unbelievable to me.

5

How Do We Select the Right Remedies?

Three principles

There are three important principles to remember when selecting remedies. The first is that we are not selecting remedies for a disease. If we have a particular illness, condition or set of symptoms we need to ignore it when we think about which remedies we need.

This can be difficult. It's natural to talk about aches and pains when people ask, 'how are you?' But in remedy terms the answers aren't useful. When you had a cold last week you might have ended up taking the same remedies as the year before, when you had a headache or a broken leg. The next time you have a cold you might need different remedies. The physical condition doesn't influence the choice. (We can of course use other forms of medicine alongside the remedies to help any immediate physical symptoms. Consult a doctor if you are worried about your physical health.)

The second principle is that we select remedies for how we feel now. The fact that we might have been unhappy or jealous or in a daydream last Tuesday is irrelevant if we don't feel that way today.

The third principle is that we aim to treat what we see. We don't need to subject ourselves to lengthy analysis in order to select remedies. Instead we can stay on the surface and select for what is obviously there. If there are deeper problems that need to be resolved these will become apparent as the remedies resolve the surface problems. (Remember the onion peeling process in Chapter 3?)

So the three principles are these:

1. Ignore physical symptoms.

2. Look at how you feel today.

3. Treat what you see.

Mood remedies

Impatience, intolerance, lack of will, apathy, self-pity, a sense of loss, discouragement, guilt, fear...all of us at different times in our lives will experience all 38 of the remedy moods. When we do, we simply pick the remedies that we need at that moment. We are using the remedies as *mood remedies*, and because we can use all 38 in this way we can say that all of the remedies are mood remedies.

Sometimes it may be enough to select and take a single remedy for a single mood. Sometimes one dose, or a couple of doses, is enough and we quickly feel better and don't have to take the remedy again.

But moods can be longer lasting, in which case they may form part of a selection of remedies designed to resolve a negative mindset. In this case, they are often mixed with one or more *type remedies*.

Type remedies

So what is a type remedy? Put simply, a type remedy is one that describes something about our fundamental character. It says how we usually react, rather than how we happen to be reacting at the moment.

We have seen that all 38 remedies can be mood remedies. When it comes to type remedies, however, the situation is different. Star of Bethlehem is for shock, Olive for tiredness and Sweet Chestnut for anguish. These and some other remedy pictures do not include descriptions of personality traits.

Examples of remedies that definitely do describe types include:

- Impatiens – for the type of person who lives life in a rush, loses patience easily and reacts to pressure by going faster.

- Beech – for the type of person who often criticises others and doesn't see value in other ways of life.

- Centaury – for the type of person who finds it hard to refuse requests for help and who is sometimes taken advantage of.

- Vine – for the type of person who will force other people to do things his way and won't take no for an answer.

These are just examples. If we read back through the remedy indications in Chapter 4 we will see many other remedies that seem to describe types of people and permanent characteristics as much as (or more than) they describe temporary moods.

In practice there is no definite, fixed list of type remedies. Some, such as Willow and Honeysuckle, inhabit a kind of grey area. They may appear to describe personalities on first reading, but almost invariably mindsets that involve self-pity, resentment and nostalgia turn out to be outer layers of the onion, with the real type hidden underneath.

What about the '12 types'?

Dr Bach's understanding of type remedies changed as he developed the system. When he had only 12 remedies – which he called 'the 12 healers' – he related each one to a fundamental personality. In the finished system most of the 12 are still described in these terms. But one in particular, Rock Rose, is no longer a type remedy – it is an emergency remedy used for terror – while the descriptions of many later remedies include personality traits.

Occasionally some writers will refer to the first 12 as 'the type remedies' but in the full system there are more than 12.

Finding your type remedy

In a sense, finding a type remedy is unimportant. As long as we follow the basic principle of treating what we see, we will always select a type remedy when we need to. Nevertheless, most people using the remedies like to take some time to work out what their type remedy might be, because the type remedy tells us something about who we are and about the main areas that we need to work on. Here are a few thought experiments that could help you think about your type remedy.

- Imagine yourself in a potentially stressful situation, such as working to a tight deadline, or taking 20 young children to the seaside for the day. How do you go about organising things? How good are you at it? What do you do when things go wrong?

- Think about your faults – or ask a friend to list them for you. What is the one thing that you need to work on most?

- Think about the qualities you admire in other people. Are they qualities that you share or qualities that you aspire to?

- Imagine you have to accompany your partner to a formal dinner where you won't know anyone. How do you feel about the prospect? How will you behave on the night?

Answering questions like these and comparing our answers with the indications for the remedies can help us get on the track of our type remedy. But we shouldn't be concerned if we remain unsure. Remembering the onion analogy and how we build up layers of emotion, there is no reason to believe we will be able to see the centre when we are peeling away the first layer. As we take remedies for successive layers, the true type remedy tends to become clearer along the way.

Can somebody's type change?

The type remedy describes our fundamental character and as such it won't change over a lifetime. That said, we may well *feel* that it changes. This is because at every layer of the onion there is the potential to be acting as if we were a different type.

Thinking back to the example of the furniture maker in Chapter 3, his type remedy when he is out of balance and losing patience with his children may appear to be Impatiens. If he stays in this state for a long time he may forget he was ever any different. As he begins to peel the onion, the Impatiens state will eventually fade. His real type may be something completely different, lying underneath: Centaury, perhaps, or Walnut or Water Violet.

Most of the time we can eventually understand people in terms of one outstanding type remedy. In some cases, however, this doesn't seem to apply, and two or more type remedies seem to be equally important – people are mixes of Mimulus and Impatiens, for example, or Vine and Vervain. In any case, the basic rule still applies. If we treat what we see, the type (or types) will eventually come into focus.

Selecting a personal mix

Selecting remedies can at first seem quite difficult. Bach practitioners often remark how new clients start off thinking they need all 38. It shouldn't be too hard though to narrow down the choice. The way to go about it is to apply the three principles that we saw at the start of this chapter:

1. Ignore physical symptoms.

2. Look at how you feel today.

3. Treat what you see.

Once we have looked through the list of remedies and made a note of the 20 or so that seem to apply, the first thing to do is strike out any that only relate to a physical symptom. We don't need to take Crab Apple (the cleansing remedy) every time we catch a cold – we only need it if the cold makes us feel contaminated and 'dirty'. Rock Water, Vervain and Beech are all associated with forms of mental rigidity, but we don't choose them just because we have a stiff neck.

Next, we can discard all the remedies that are for the way we felt last week or last night. That leaves those that relate to the way we feel now.

Then we can take out any that are based on guesswork. We only want to include remedies for what we can see. So if we think that there might be some shock in our background that explains our current unhappiness, but we can't actually identify what the shock might have been, then we don't need to include Star of Bethlehem. If the shock is really there and really relevant it will appear more clearly once we have taken the initial mix of remedies.

Ideally we should take no more than six or seven remedies at a time. So what do we do if we have applied these principles and still seem to have too many in our list?

The answer is to rank the remedies in order of importance. For example, you might have chosen Vine because you recognise yourself in that description. You have certainly been laying down the law for the past few days and you were a bit like that as a child as well. Perhaps it is even your type remedy. And you may have chosen Gentian because you felt a bit down in the mouth first thing this morning when you burnt the toast. Although both remedies relate to today, Vine is more important than Gentian. You can discard the Gentian.

By applying this criterion to all the remedies on your list, you should be able to isolate those that are most important to you at this moment and get the number down.

Should I always include my type remedy?

Because our type remedy describes who we are and how we tend to react when things go wrong, we usually end up including it in our mix. Does this mean that it is a good idea to always include our type remedy?

The short answer is, no. The same criterion applies as when selecting any other remedy: we only need to include our type remedy if we are in that negative state right now. Imagine your type remedy is Vervain: you are naturally enthusiastic and energetic, and sometimes your enthusiasm goes too far. There would be no point taking Vervain if you found yourself in a Hornbeam state, or today is one of your rare Wild Rose days.

Even when mixing a treatment bottle – which we tend to do for longer-term issues – there will be times when our type remedy is not involved in how we feel. If it isn't needed, there is no need to take it.

What if I need a remedy that is not in the system?

Dr Bach believed that the system was complete, which means that it contains a remedy for every possible negative mental state that a human being can feel. How can this be true? Surely there are more than 38 negative states? And what do we do if we feel something that doesn't seem to be covered by one of the 38?

One way to explore these questions is to draw an analogy with colour. Computers can display millions of colours – but there are an infinite number of gradations and human eyes normally distinguish many more. Yet all we see can be reproduced by mixing just three primary colours: red, blue and yellow.

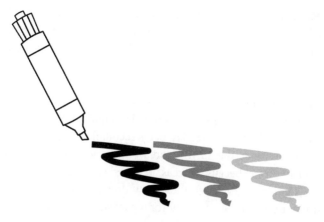

Figure 5.1 Three colours combined
can colour the universe

In the same way, human beings can feel an infinite number of different shades of emotion. Yet all of them can be reproduced using a combination of just 38 basic states, and for every one of those basic states there is a remedy in Dr Bach's system.

Based on there being 39 remedies (38 plus the emergency mix, which is usually thought of as a separate remedy) and an absolute maximum of nine remedies in a mix (Dr Bach twice gave this number), there are nearly 293 million available combinations.

Furthermore, two different people who need the same remedies usually need them for slightly different reasons. George and his work colleague Jemima might both need Impatiens and Mimulus, but their reasons for taking them could be different. Perhaps George is an Impatiens type who has agreed at once to speak at a conference without thinking it through. He hasn't had time to prepare, and now he is anxious about what will happen. Jemima might be a Mimulus type who is dreading the conference because it will mean having to meet lots of strangers afterwards. She needs Impatiens because her anxiety is making her more impatient than usual with her children.

The fact that an apparently identical mix of remedies can cover different mentalities supports the claim that 38 remedies are enough. And there is empirical evidence as well: The Bach Centre has been recommending remedies to people since the 1930s, and we have never had to send someone away because there is no remedy for their condition.

On a practical level, then, how do we cope when there doesn't seem to be a remedy for a particular problem?

The answer is to break down the emotion to find out what it really means. For example, you may be suffering from stress. There is no remedy for stress *per se*, so you need to find out what stress means to you and why it is there.

Are you stressed because you are trying to do everything too fast (Impatiens) or because you feel unfulfilled and can't find anything worthwhile to do (Wild Oat)? Are you putting yourself under stress by throwing yourself into a project (Vervain) or are you stressed because you have allowed someone else to control your life (Centaury)?

Similarly, there is no one remedy for anger. So if you are feeling angry you need to start by identifying the cause – intolerant Beech, spiteful Holly, indignant Vervain or resentful Willow – before you can select the right remedies.

The same thing applies to any feeling we have that doesn't seem to be covered: with a little thought we can quickly identify the remedies we need.

6

How Do We Take Remedies?

For passing moods

It's Monday. You come home after a day's work feeling tired, and you snap at the children for making too much noise. You need to take some Olive and Beech to help you out of this mood so you can enjoy your evening. Here's how to do it.

1. Put some water in a glass.

2. Add two drops of Beech and two drops of Olive.

3. Sip from the glass until you feel better.

If you were including Dr Bach's emergency formula in the glass you would add four drops of that remedy – the amount doubles because it is a combination. You don't need to worry about the size of the glass or the amount of water in it. Two drops from a single stock bottle is well above the minimum needed for a regular-sized glass, so there is plenty of margin for error.

You could put the drops into something other than water if you prefer. Bach remedies are much more robust than classical homoeopathic medicines, so you can add them to coffee, tea, beer or food without any concern.

On the whole, the remedies work quickly in this sort of situation, and sipping a few drops diluted in a drink is perhaps the easiest way to prevent negative emotions from hanging around too long.

Mixing a treatment bottle

What if you are dealing with a more long-term problem and need to take the same mix of remedies for several days or weeks?

You can, if you want, use the same system: just mix the remedies in a glass of water and sip from it throughout the day (at least four times during the day). Then you make up a fresh glass each morning. But there is another method that is more economical and easier in the long run: to make up a treatment bottle.

A treatment bottle is a small medicine bottle containing water and the remedies that you want to take. Here is what to do.

1. Get an empty 30 ml (one ounce) dropper bottle (a dropper bottle is a bottle with a pipette built into the lid; you should be able to get one from the same place that you buy remedies). If you can't get a 30 ml bottle any smaller size will do.

2. Put two drops of each selected remedy into the bottle (and four drops of the emergency mix if you are including that).

3. Top up with mineral water – use the non-gassy kind so that it doesn't spill over the top.

From this mixed treatment bottle you need to take four drops, at least four times a day. Ideally you would space the doses out, taking the first one on waking and the last before you go to bed. You can take four-drop doses more often if you need to.

To take the remedies from the treatment bottle, drop the drops straight onto your tongue. Some people prefer to drop them under the tongue. You can also take them via a teaspoon of water or add them to tea, coffee or fruit juice – as long as you get the four-drop dose into you.

Treatment bottles are useful because they are easy to carry around. We can take a dose of our personal mix whenever we want, quickly and easily. We save money as well, because we end up using much less remedy than we would if we were making up remedies in a glass each day.

A 30 ml treatment bottle will last up to three weeks, assuming we take the drops regularly. To keep the water fresh for that long we can keep the bottle in the fridge, or include a teaspoon of brandy (or any similar strength spirit) when we first mix it together. With or without the brandy, mineral water keeps best. Tap water deteriorates more quickly even if we boil it first. Distilled water should not be used, as it is biologically dead.

By the way, sometimes people assume that Bach remedies should not be stored in fridges. There is in fact no evidence that they are affected by the electromagnetic fields generated by household appliances, TVs and computers.

If you get a couple of days into your treatment bottle and realise you need an additional remedy, just add it to the mix – assuming this doesn't mean you will be taking more than seven or so remedies at a time. Where adding remedies would take you over that limit, you might be better off discarding the treatment bottle and starting again. For the purpose of counting the number of remedies in a mix, the emergency combination counts as just one remedy.

Can we re-use treatment bottles?

Even if you add brandy to a treatment bottle *and* keep it in the fridge, sooner or later the water will go off. Every time you open the bottle you are giving bacteria a chance to get into the liquid. If the dropper touches your tongue this is almost certain to happen.

We can re-use treatment bottles, but because of the risk of contamination it is a good idea to sterilise them first. To do this, remove all the plastic and rubber parts and place the glass (the dropper and the bottle itself) into a saucepan of water. The glass dropper should pull out of the rubber top quite easily. Heat the saucepan and bring to the boil, and allow it to bubble for between 15 and 20 minutes. Remove the glassware and leave it to dry naturally, or for a sparkling finish place the bottles upside down in a warm oven.

The plastic top and rubber teat can be washed in hot water. It is best not to boil them unless absolutely necessary, as eventually this will damage them.

An alternative to boiling is to use one of the systems designed for sterilising babies' bottles. A steam steriliser is the best solution. Sterilising tablets are less good because they leave a residue in the bottles, which will give your next mix a chemical taste.

In an emergency

In an emergency there is no time to make up treatment bottles and there may not even be time to find a glass of water. In this case we can take undiluted drops straight from a stock bottle. (Stock bottles are the concentrated remedies on sale in the shops.) The dosage is two drops on the tongue, or four of the combination crisis remedy, repeated as necessary.

What if someone has fainted and is unable to swallow? In this situation we could apply the remedies to pulse points on the neck, wrist or temple. This is not as efficient as taking them by mouth in the usual way, but the effects will still be felt.

Other uses

The remedies are designed to be ingested and the best results are achieved using that method. Sometimes, however, people like to use them in other ways, usually as a backup to taking them orally. The commonest techniques include using the remedies:

- in compresses
- as a lotion
- in the bath
- in sprays.

Dr Bach was a fan of compresses, as we saw in Chapter 4. To make up a compress, dilute two drops of each selected remedy (four of the crisis mix) into a small bowl of water. Use ice-cold water for swollen areas (you can add ice cubes as well if you want) and warm water for stiffened muscles and so on. Take a clean cloth, wet it in the medicated water and apply to the affected area.

For a lotion of remedies, put two drops of each remedy into a glass of water, as you would if you were going to sip from it. Then bathe the affected area in the water or dab the liquid on using a clean cotton-wool ball. This kind of use can be built into a regular cleansing routine if you are troubled with a skin problem.

Some people find that adding remedies to the bath can have a beneficial and relaxing effect. There is no exact dosage for this: three or four drops of each individual remedy should do, and double the amount of the crisis mix if that is what you are using.

Finally, you could add remedies to a water mister (the kind used to spray plants) and use this to freshen the room. A couple of drops of single remedies and four of the crisis mix should be sufficient.

All of these methods have been found useful, and one remedy maker now produces the crisis mix in a ready-to-use spray. But it should be stressed once again that they are secondary to taking the remedies by mouth. That remains the quickest, simplest and most effective way of using them.

How fast do the remedies work?

Answering this question is like trying to say how long it takes to climb a mountain: it depends on the climber and the size of the mountain. Nevertheless, there are some general rules to guide us.

First of all, and as we might expect, the remedies tend to work faster on moods than on deep-rooted issues. This is one reason there are more dramatic stories told about the crisis mix than about any of the single remedies. We use the crisis formula for emergencies, i.e. outside events that have thrown us off course. Usually the remedies can quickly correct these immediate imbalances and get us back to where we were.

Despite the occasional story of sudden cures and immediate relief, in general the more deep-seated imbalances – the kind for which we would normally want to make up a treatment bottle – take longer to resolve. This is because they have taken root in us – sometimes so much so that they seem to have become part of our personality. The more deep-rooted they are, the longer the treatment.

Nevertheless, we would normally expect to see some improvement after three weeks, even in longstanding conditions. When nothing happens we can take this as a cue to look again at the selection of remedies to see if it is as appropriate as we thought it was. Three weeks is about the time that a treatment bottle will last, so this is a natural time to review a selection.

Often we barely notice improvements until we look for them. Balance tends to be less visible than imbalance, just as we don't notice being well in the same way that we notice being ill. We can think of nothing else when we have a headache, but when the headache goes we forget it and get on with our lives. We may only realise how far we have come when we think back to how things were before we started taking the remedies. Some people say that their friends notice a change before they do. Comments like 'you're looking well' or 'you seem cheerful today' can be the first clue we have that negativity and stress have melted away.

Allergies and reactions

People suffering from allergies occasionally ask if they too will be able to use the remedies safely. Someone with an intolerance for aspirin might wonder if the Willow remedy is safe, as the salicin used in aspirin came originally from the bark and leaves of the willow tree. Others might worry about taking Walnut if they are allergic to nuts.

We saw in the first chapter of this book that each remedy is made using the plant named on the bottle. But once the flowering parts have energised the water, remedy makers remove the plant material, and stock remedies contain only very small amounts of the resulting mother tincture. Chemical analysis shows that there is no plant-derived material in a stock bottle at all, and this is why people with allergies to the plants don't need to worry about using the remedies.

In fact, the only genuine safety concern is that stock remedies are bottled and preserved in alcohol. We will look at that in more depth at the end of this chapter.

If the remedies don't cause allergies, what about reactions – in other words, negative or harmful effects? The short answer is that they don't cause reactions either, at least not in the way most orthodox drugs do. Bach remedies re-energise our positive emotions – they are wholly beneficial in their effect.

There is a longer answer, though, and it helps to explain why people sometimes complain that the remedies have caused not a state of balance but a different (or greater) state of imbalance.

As we saw in Chapter 3, dealing with deep-rooted problems may involve working back through several layers of negative state before the fundamental imbalance is revealed. Someone who is taking Scleranthus for her indecisiveness may begin to feel critical of the people around her and blame this on the remedy. What is happening is that the layer of indecisiveness is being cleansed, and underlying feelings of intolerance, which may have been pushed away and hidden for many years, are showing. The remedies haven't made the person intolerant – they have just revealed that there is intolerance there.

The answer to developments like this is to select further remedies to deal with the newly revealed negative states. In our example, we might suggest Beech either as well as or instead of Scleranthus.

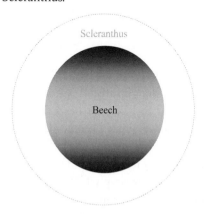

Figure 6.1 Buried emotions may come to the surface as the first layer is dealt with

A similar situation can arise when someone takes remedies and finds that the negative emotions seem to get stronger rather than weaker. This happens when the remedy helps to bring feelings more into our consciousness. Taking remedies makes us more aware of how we feel, so that it can seem as if things are worse simply because we are more aware of them. The answer, again, is to persevere. The remedies are only and always positive in their effect. Increased consciousness of a problem is the first step to resolving it.

Finally, and in extremely rare cases, some people experience what appear to be physical reactions to the remedies. They can take the form of minor rashes, headaches or rises in body temperature. In all cases symptoms are mild and don't last long. They can be understood as the physical signs of an emotional cleansing. If you experience more pronounced symptoms, or your symptoms go on longer than a day or so, this has nothing to do with the remedies. You should consult a qualified medical practitioner.

Don't let this talk of reactions put you off using Dr Bach's system. It is the safest and most gentle form of medicine around – so much so that Bach remedies can be given (suitably diluted) even to newborn babies. We can use them without fear.

When should we stop taking remedies?

The answer is quite straightforward. We stop taking remedies when we no longer feel that we need them. They are not habit-forming and we won't become dependent on them, so we don't have to wean ourselves off by reducing doses gradually. In fact many people find that when they no longer need their remedies they simply forget to take them.

Sometimes people continue to take drops because they are concerned that the negative feelings may come back. This isn't something to worry about. The remedies work to strengthen our positive emotions and once they are strengthened they remain strong. It's a bit like mending a broken fence: we don't have to keep hammering once the fence is strong, because it can stand by itself. If in a week's time a hurricane should come and blow the fence down, that's time enough to start mending it again. In other words, if something happens to throw you back out of balance then – and only then – you can go back to the remedies. They are always there to help.

In truth, ideal use of the remedies involves a continuous relationship with them. Once we have resolved any treatment-bottle-scale problems, we can still use the system as mood remedies to keep us in balance whatever life throws at us. This was Dr Bach's vision for the future: 'I want to make it as simple as this,' he said, 'I am hungry, I will go and pull a lettuce from the garden for my tea; I am frightened and ill, I will take a dose of Mimulus.'

A note on alcohol

As we saw when we looked at the methods used to prepare remedies, remedy makers use brandy as a preservative and as a liquid carrying medium for the energised water. We saw that a 10 ml stock bottle of remedy contains two-thirds of a drop of mother tincture, while the rest is usually 27 per cent or 40 per cent proof brandy. This can be a worry to parents who want to give remedies to their children. It causes a particular problem for people who have decided not to take alcohol for health or religious reasons.

Parents at least will be reassured when they understand how much alcohol is actually in a dose. A treatment bottle is 30 ml of water plus just two drops of each selected remedy. A dose from this bottle is only four drops. The amount of alcohol in a dose of that size is barely measurable, especially when compared with the quantity of alcohol that occurs naturally in many foods. A glass of orange juice could contain as much as 0.4 per cent ABV (alcohol by volume) – yet even at this level, which is much greater than in a Bach flower remedy dose, the body metabolises the alcohol as fast as we take it in. Four drops from a treatment bottle is not going to intoxicate anybody.

The same considerations, however, may not help adults with religious objections to alcohol. Some religions will make special dispensation for medical use. If you feel this might apply you need to ask your spiritual advisor for guidance. Orthodox Jews have a particular problem in that most remedies are not kosher. Advice on this issue should be sought from a rabbi. Where taking drops by mouth would not be possible, the rules might allow you to use the remedies externally, applying them to the temples or wrists or other pulse points.

Using the remedies externally can be an option for recovering alcoholics as well. Another solution is to put the treatment bottle drops into a very hot drink, which will evaporate the trace alcohol.

Special mention needs to be made of a group of drugs that are sometimes given to recovering alcoholics to help them stop drinking. The most common of these – disulfiram – is marketed as Antabuse. Disulfiram reacts to the presence of alcohol and causes the person who has taken it to feel extremely ill. Some reports suggest that the use of alcohol-based aftershaves has caused reactions in susceptible people who have taken Antabuse. This makes the external use of remedies problematic and the best advice is to speak to the person who prescribed the drug in the first place.

Some people who have stopped drinking feel able to use the remedies when they find out how dilute a treatment bottle dose is. Others are more nervous. People who have sworn never to drink again can feel that taking in even a trace amount represents the breaking of a promise. The psychological impact in such cases could be out of all proportion to the amount of alcohol involved. Many alcohol counsellors advise their clients not to use alcohol-based Bach remedies.

In all cases where the alcohol content of the remedies is a problem the final decision must be left in the hands of the individual concerned. All of us who use them to help others have a duty to be clear about the alcohol content so that people can make an informed decision.

Alcohol-free remedies

In recent years some remedy makers have started to supply selected remedies in alcohol-free formulations. The starting point is still a mother tincture made with brandy, but instead of being diluted into further brandy the stock bottle liquid is a mix of glycerine and water, or a preservative based on fruit or vinegar. The trace levels of alcohol in the stock bottles means they would be classed as 'alcohol-free' under UK food regulations.

Once these stock remedies are diluted into a treatment bottle the amount of alcohol in a dose is effectively zero. A chemical analysis would not find any alcohol in four drops from a treatment bottle made with an alcohol-free stock remedy.

7

How Can We Help Others?

Learning the remedies

If we want to help others with the remedies the first priority is to learn the system well. This may sound obvious, but in fact most of us tend to learn best the four or five remedies that we take most often. When we start to help other people we pick up on the slightest indication for these remedies and often miss more obvious selections from among the remaining 34 or so.

In my role as a teacher of the system I often see evidence of this in the classroom and in written work. One person sees Larch everywhere because that is the remedy he is taking. Another feels himself surrounded by Vine types. A third believes that everybody needs Agrimony.

How does one learn the remedies well? Reading this book is a help, obviously, but reading alone is not enough. We need to start thinking with the remedies. Ideally the various categories, types and moods should be as familiar to us as the terms extrovert and introvert are to a psychologist, or ego, id and super-ego to a psychoanalyst. We know the system really well when we are able to classify people under remedy headings in the same way we classify colours into red, green, blue, yellow and orange.

At the moment this may sound like a faint and faraway ideal, but we can get close to it surprisingly quickly if we take the trouble to build the remedies into our everyday lives.

For example, most of us watch television drama from time to time. Drama has to be dramatic, and the lives of fictional characters on television are often wholly out of balance. They spend every waking moment lurching from one crisis to another.

We can take advantage of this. Next time you watch television try to pinpoint the type and mood remedies that the characters on the screen might need. Pay attention to what they say and the things they do, and to the way the actors use facial expression, body posture and mannerisms to communicate character and emotion. What you see is a mirror of the way real people communicate in real life, using words, tone of voice, body language and gesture.

We can do the same thing with characters in films, plays and novels, and with personalities from history, people in the news and people we meet in everyday life. Most of our acquaintances are probably not as emotionally transparent as the members of a soap opera family so this last may seem slightly more difficult. But we are not attempting a deep analysis of every acquaintance. We are simply noticing things and applying the system of 38 remedies to our observations. The important thing is to get into the habit of thinking with the remedies.

To avoid the trap of reading your own remedies into the people around you, refer frequently to the remedy indications and try to be more exact in your choices. Is so-and-so really Centaury, as your intuition tells you? Or would Wild Rose or Walnut be more appropriate? To decide, imagine the same person if she were an out-and-out Wild Rose or Walnut – how close to the real person is your caricature?

We can use the same technique when we find it hard to learn a remedy, or to remember the differences between particular pairs of remedies: Larch and Elm, for example, which are both for lack of confidence, or Gentian and Gorse for degrees of discouragement, or Scleranthus and Wild Oat for varieties of indecision. Imagine a person in a situation, such as attending a job interview and ask yourself how he would feel and react if he needed first Larch, then Elm, then Scleranthus, then Wild Oat.

Let's try that now. In a Larch state the interviewee would be convinced that he was going to fail. Being so convinced, he might not try very hard to succeed. He might even decide not to turn up at all. In an Elm state the same person would feel quite capable of doing the job and deep down would know his own abilities. He would go to the interview, but on hearing the extent of the responsibilities that go with the job he might become concerned about whether he could take them on in addition to all the other things that he is already committed to. His would be a crisis of confidence caused by the prospect of additional responsibilities; the Larch reaction would be a chronic lack of confidence that causes him to avoid taking responsibility in the first place.

In a Scleranthus state, the interviewee wouldn't be sure whether to take the job or not. First he would think, yes, it sounds good, just what I need, then at once he would reconsider. Maybe he should stay where he is? Does he want to commute this far out, or should he maybe try to find a similar job closer to home?

In a Wild Oat state the doubt would lie at a deeper level. He would be somebody looking for a career with a meaning. He would want to achieve something special, something fulfilling. He isn't sure what direction to go in, so the question is, does this job offer true fulfilment? He isn't sure, but he will probably accept it rather than stay where he is – his current position has brought nothing but frustration.

Imagining people in situations like this is an excellent way to improve our knowledge and get to know all 38 flower remedies on a more intimate level. When we come to select remedies for other people the insight gained in such games will prove invaluable.

Improving your selection skills

This book can't teach you how to be a practitioner. Nevertheless, some of the skills that a practitioner calls on can be useful when we try to help friends and family. The first and most important is to listen to what is being said. This should be obvious, but many of us find it difficult. We start thinking about what we are going to say next, or about how we felt when the same thing once happened to us.

Knowing the remedies really well helps us to listen. If we are trying to work out the subtle difference between Gentian and Gorse while our friend is saying that she might as well give up, we are probably going to miss any clues that indicate a different remedy entirely.

A related point is to remember *why* we are listening. If we become too interested in people's stories we risk forgetting that our focus should be on their feelings. On courses we talk about moving from story to feelings to remedies: listening to a story is just a stage on the way to understanding emotions. We can't get too wrapped up in what happened next or what one person said to another; still less use the story by itself as a way to select remedies. People don't need Walnut because they have moved house – it's how they feel about the move that indicates perhaps Walnut, perhaps something else.

Another useful practitioner skill is the ability to leave a silence. If our friend stops talking for a moment but is obviously collecting her thoughts we don't need to jump straight in with a question. It can be better to wait and allow her the time she needs to work things out in her mind.

If we do ask questions, we should be careful not to direct people towards the answers we want or expect. For example, a friend might say she feels tired. Maybe she needs Hornbeam or Olive? If we ask a question like 'Are you tired first thing in the morning or last thing at night?' or 'Do you get tired at the end of the day?' we are not leaving her any room to talk more about how she actually feels. We are pushing her down a particular path, and it should be no surprise that we will get confirmation of our selection more often than not, and give her either Hornbeam or Olive.

Rather than ask closed questions like these it's better to ask open questions – questions that can't be answered with a 'yes' or 'no', and that don't restrict the range of possible answers. Open questions tend to begin with the words 'what', 'when', 'who', 'why' or 'how'. So we might ask our tired-looking friend something like, 'What sort of things make you feel tired?', 'When do you get tired?' or, 'How do you feel right now?' Each of these gives her space to choose her own response.

Another leaf from the good practitioner's book is to try to share our knowledge of the remedies so as to involve our friend in the selection process. Asking open questions goes some way towards this. We can go further by explaining which remedies we are considering and telling our friend what they are for. That way she has an opportunity to learn some of the indications herself, can decide which of the suggested remedies is closest to how she feels and can disagree with our choice if she feels we have got it wrong.

Sometimes we may feel reluctant to explain a choice. It can be particularly awkward if we are thinking about remedies whose indications are less than flattering. Few of us would mind hearing that Larch and White Chestnut mean we are a bit lacking in confidence and inclined to worry too much, but how would we feel knowing that Heather,

Willow and Beech mean that we are considered to be self-pitying, intolerant bores?

Explaining the remedies certainly calls for a measure of tact. There are a few well-worn techniques that can help. For a start, we can stress that all the remedy states are normal, everyday human emotions and that all of us feel these things from time to time. Then we could explain what a remedy is for by giving an example of when we ourselves used it. (But keep the example short. We don't want to hog the stage and start telling stories of our own.)

We could also relate the choice of a remedy back to the things our friend said during the conversation. For example, she might have mentioned that her husband is getting on her nerves. We could remind her of this and say that Beech is a remedy to help us cope better with people and behaviours that annoy us.

Finally, we can stress the positive aspect of the remedies. Look back through the remedy indications in Chapter 4 and you will see that every remedy has its positive aspect. We might explain the selection of Heather, then, by talking about how it helps us look beyond our immediate concerns and how it gets our problems back into perspective.

If you follow these basic rules you will be well on your way to helping others. Once the word gets out that you have had a success with a friend or a relation, don't be surprised when more requests for help come your way.

Selecting for younger children

People sometimes assume that it must be difficult to select remedies for younger children. This is a pity in many ways. Perhaps because their true feelings are closer to the surface and they haven't yet learned to conceal what they feel from the outside world, and from themselves, children can respond very quickly to the remedies.

It is in fact fairly easy in most cases to select remedies for children, even when they are too young to explain how they feel. One can even select for babies who can barely communicate at all. The key is observation and empathy.

To start with, we can spend time with the child while he is playing and look at how he reacts. Is he short-tempered or patient? Does he like to spend a long time absorbed in one activity or does he go from one thing to another? If he falls over or hurts himself, how does he behave? Putting these clues together we can soon come up with a list of possible choices, and because the remedies are harmless there is no danger involved if we end up choosing the wrong ones. The worst that can happen is that the mix will have no effect.

For small children, some remedies are much more used than others. The crisis formula is a favourite, because it's always near at hand for accidents and upsets. Walnut is another useful remedy to keep in the nursery: it helps unsettled children get used to the stages they go through in the early years, from being born to getting teeth to weaning to starting school. For the inevitable temper tantrums you could try Cherry Plum.

The dosage for children is the same as for adults. For very small babies four drops from a treatment bottle (prepared using cooled, boiled water) can be added to a milk feed. Or you might prefer to stroke remedies onto the top of a baby's head. If mum is breastfeeding she can take the mix herself and the effects will pass to the baby through the breast milk. For older children you can mix the drops in with food or fruit juice.

A practitioner's story

Louise, William's mother, phoned me for an appointment. She said she got my telephone number from another mum she met at the baby clinic. Her GP was against complementary therapies and referred to them as 'mumbo-jumbo' and 'a load of rubbish', but she said she was so desperate she would try anything.

I could hear William screaming as I parked my car and walked up the path to the front door. Louise looked totally exhausted – eyes red with dark rings underneath, very pale, hair not brushed and wearing a dressing-gown at two o'clock in the afternoon. She apologised for the untidy state of the house and offered me a cup of tea, saying she hadn't had a chance to make one for herself that day. I accepted and held William while she made it. William continued to scream very loudly. He was rigid and stiff and made constant, jerky movements with his arms, legs and head. He seemed very hot and looked very red.

I introduced Louise to the remedies and explained their gentle and benign action. Conversation was very difficult due to William's screaming, interspersed with little coughs, but I asked Louise about her pregnancy.

She had gone through a difficult time, always throwing up, and had spent the second and third months in bed as a miscarriage was feared. The hospital had assured her that William had been unaffected by all this. When asked, she said that William had kicked and moved around a lot, 'almost as if he couldn't wait to get out and get on with it.'

The birth had been straightforward but Louise said that William began to splutter, cry and yell almost immediately and could not be pacified. He kept the whole maternity wing awake until a private room was made available. Louise chose to bottle-feed William and found he was very difficult to feed as he just took gulps in between screams and coughed most of it up again. It all took a long time and he was slightly underweight.

I asked Louise about the rest of the family. She already has one daughter and had no problems with her as a baby. Her daughter hadn't taken to William, as the crying and screaming kept her awake at night. She was falling asleep at school.

She felt he had disrupted everything and that he didn't want to be cuddled or loved. As for Louise's partner he worked long hours to make ends meet, and couldn't stand William's constant screaming. He had gone to stay with his mother and only returned for clean clothes.

Throughout our conversation William continued to scream loudly except for two occasions when, utterly exhausted, he fell into a brief and fitful sleep, in which he twitched, moved and whimpered. Almost as soon as he dozed off he coughed, which woke him up, and the screaming began again. Louise said that the longest span he had slept since birth was 1 hour and 35 minutes. He could not be pacified or comforted, remained very stiff (while asleep as well as awake) and I felt he would prefer to be left alone rather than be held or fussed. Louise confirmed this.

The cough was not dry, but sounded like mucus in the throat, not on the chest. It had been there since birth. Her GP said it was due to his not having his airways sucked out properly in the delivery room and said he would probably grow out of it at around age six months. If he didn't, something would then be done.

Louise told me that she was unable to go out at all as people stared at William. No one was willing to babysit for him, and she relied on her daughter for shopping. Neighbours had complained about the noise.

I considered which remedies were required. I decided on Crab Apple for its cleansing properties, Olive for his total exhaustion, Impatiens for his irritation and his wanting to be left alone and Cherry Plum for his loss of control – he seemed at the end of his tether.

Other remedies that crossed my mind but that I decided against were Vervain (the fretting was not of this nature), Water Violet (there was a need to be left alone, but this was more Impatiens in nature), Rock Water (there was physical rigidity, but it was more connected with Impatiens and Cherry Plum), Star of Bethlehem (there were no known shocks or birth traumas) and Walnut (I felt his adjustment to life was not a major consideration).

I felt Impatiens could be his type remedy, as it was indicated even before birth.

I explained all the chosen remedies to Louise and she agreed with all the indications except she was convinced that the crab apples in their garden were poisonous. I did my best to convince her otherwise but she phoned her father to check. The father confirmed that crab apples were quite safe but then began to shout at her for having some quack in the house and told her not to let me anywhere near the baby. I could hear this from across the room.

I gave William back to Louise so I could mix up the remedies and explained the dose and that it should be administered in a little cooled, boiled water. While I did this Louise changed William and tried to feed him. There was no change in his behaviour. I made sure that Louise still had my telephone number, emphasised again the benign action of the remedies and tried to give her reassurance and instil hope and confidence in the remedies. William continued to scream.

I felt I'd built up a reasonable rapport, considering that Louise was very wary and suspicious – even a little hostile – at first. I left after one-and-a-half hours feeling I needed some remedies myself and a lie down in a darkened room; I could still hear William screaming as I got into my car.

When I arrived home about three-quarters of an hour later there was a hysterical message on my answering machine from Louise, wanting me to call back at once. William was very ill! What had I done to him?

I phoned straight back. Louise had given William his first dose, and he'd stopped crying almost immediately and fallen asleep. I explained that this was the best we could hope for, tried to calm her, explained again that the remedies are totally harmless. Louise was still very upset and angry, convinced I'd poisoned her baby.

A few days later Louise phoned again. After her last call to me, she bundled William into a blanket and ran with him to her GP's surgery. A locum doctor had assured her that William was just sleeping, albeit very deeply. He encouraged her to continue with the remedies as all else had failed. William slept until 10pm, when Louise woke him to be fed. She gave him a second dose of remedies at the same time; he cried a little but was soon asleep again. He slept until 2am, when Louise panicked and woke him once more. He coughed a little but didn't cry. She was so worried she called her GP's number and the locum doctor visited at around 3am. He was quite cross and said, again, that William was absolutely OK. Not convinced, an hour later she carried William to the casualty department at the local hospital, where he was pronounced to be fine. One of the nurses there said that she used the remedies and Louise was very much reassured by this and decided to continue with William's treatment.

During the ensuing week, William's cough had steadily improved and was now gone. He had settled into a routine, sleeping 12 hours each night, and being woken at 10pm to be fed. He was now feeding well. Sometimes he cried a little but the screaming had stopped completely, and he slept peacefully without jerking or being rigid. Louise's partner had moved back, a neighbour had offered to babysit from time to time and her daughter had brought a school friend to meet William.

When I visited by appointment a few weeks later I was amazed at the change in William and absolutely thrilled to see him so calm and content. His remedies were used up and Louise asked for some more. I felt that the Crab Apple, Cherry Plum and Olive were no longer required, but I put a couple of drops of Impatiens into a treatment bottle as I felt it might be a good idea to continue with his type remedy for a little longer. A couple of weeks later, when the bottle ran out, I said I felt he didn't need the remedies any more, that they had done their work. Louise got very agitated, worried that William's problems would return. After much reassurance from me that everything would be fine and she could always call me if it wasn't, she agreed to see how William got on without the remedies.

Over the next couple of months several of Louise's friends contacted me, having been referred by her, and when I bumped into her and the rest of the family next it was at the railway station. They had just returned from a weekend away and William had coped with a long, crowded train journey with no problems. He still slept well, the cough hadn't returned, and he remained relaxed and well balanced.

I was quite surprised at how quickly William returned from such an extreme state to a state of equilibrium. Now I have had more experience with babies I know that they do seem to respond very quickly. It was a great privilege to work with William and I can't help smiling every time I think of the brilliant outcome thanks to Dr Bach's remedies.

Helping animals

The problems involved in selecting remedies for small children are magnified when we try to select for animals. This is probably why people turn to the crisis mix so often and to the rest of the system so rarely. Yet given a little thought and study, it is possible to make a more focused choice.

The best way to start is to consider what life looks like to the species we are dealing with. Different species see things differently from us and differently from each other. We need, if possible, to understand their point of view so as to assess sensibly the possible emotional causes of their behaviour. In the case of domesticated animals we also need to factor in the effect of living with humans. Adapting to our rules and expectations can in itself push animals into a state of imbalance.

Take dogs as an example. We used to think that canine societies were hierarchical. The strongest and most aggressive animal in a group would be the pack leader. The weakest would be at the bottom. Every dog knew its place. Research into the lives of wild wolves at the end of the 1990s by David Mech of the University of Minnesota suggested that this understanding was probably wrong. Rather than linear dominance, it is now thought that the key factors that influence social interaction in canines are co-operation, consensus and relationships between parents and offspring.

There is an ongoing argument about the extent to which we can apply the results of studies on wolves to the behaviour of domestic dogs, but if anything dogs might in some ways be even more socially and emotionally intelligent than their wild cousins. One study in 2008 found that dogs know how to look at human faces for emotional cues. Their eyes flick left so as to scan the right side of the face – the side that shows our feelings and intentions most clearly. No other species has been found to do this. Even more fascinating, dogs don't look at other dogs or other animals in this way. Far from seeing us as members of their pack, they know we are a different species and have worked out how to read us.

What does this tell us in remedy terms? One thing it should do is make us less likely to assume that every failed interaction between dog and human is down to an ongoing struggle for dominance. Our relationships with dogs are not the Vine versus Vine confrontations some owners assume. They are far more nuanced. Furthermore, knowing that dogs are scanning our faces to see how we feel, we could be right to assume that our moods affect them much more than we once suspected. It could be a good idea to select remedies for ourselves and our dogs at the same time. The real issue might be our emotions, not theirs.

Add to this that a natural time for dogs to be active is the early mornings, just as we are leaving for work and leaving them behind, and we have a further insight into the reasons our dog might whine, chew furniture and generally misbehave when he is left alone for the day. We are more likely to choose helpful remedies – and find other helpful solutions – when we assume anxiety, frustration, boredom and loneliness are what this intelligent social creature feels. We are less likely to be right if we assume he is attacking our shoes because he is spiteful and vindictive, or trying to get one over on us.

From dogs, we turn to cats. The most common mistake we make with cats is to assume that they are solitary, haughty creatures that prefer to live alone. Many remedy users give Water Violet to felines almost as a matter of course. In fact the lifestyle of domestic cats – assuming they have the freedom to live how they choose – is not at all solitary. They generally hunt alone, but in other respects they enjoy a rich social life in a network of stable relationships. Cats sleep, play and even raise kittens together. Their social network extends geographically into a series of territories and home patches. Territories overlap. As well as having their own areas, cats negotiate rights of way over the territories of others. It is no wonder, then, if our cat seems distressed and unsettled when we move house. He has been uprooted not just from a familiar house and garden but also from all his social ties and habits.

Dogs and cats are both predators so they have characteristics in common with us and with each other – not least, forward-pointing eyes designed to lock onto prey and gauge distances. The world of prey animals like rabbits and horses is very different. In the wild, being picked up by a large predator would be the last thing a rabbit experienced before being eaten. So it would almost certainly be a mistake to choose Vine for a rabbit that bites us when we try to cuddle it. Mimulus and Rock Rose are far more likely to be useful. Many prey animals have eyes on the sides of their heads so they can see predators approaching from any angle. They use speed to escape. With this in mind, we can appreciate that a mare living in a stable could be very unhappy. She can't see what's coming – the walls are in the way – and she can't run away from noises because the door is shut. An environment that seems safe and secure to predators like us is to her an alien, threatening place.

These examples show how learning about the natural history of a species can help us understand its mental and emotional outlook. Things to look for include information on social behaviour (do they live in groups, like rabbits, or alone, like hamsters?), feeding habits (do they hunt or are they hunted?) and sex differences (how do males and females behave?).

But this is just a start. Knowing about a species only tells us what its response to a particular situation is likely to be. Individual reactions still depend on the individual personality of the animal. This is why it is easier by far to select remedies for an animal that lives with us as one of the family. Most of us know something about the personalities of the animals in our home. It is much more difficult when the animal concerned lives outside. Sheep number 38 is going to be more of an enigma, even for the farmer.

All we can do in such cases is look at the animal and ask ourselves how it compares with the average for its species. Is it particularly curious, or surprisingly fond of its own company, for a sheep? Are there other unusual behavioural quirks that make it stand out from the crowd? If it is under stress for some reason, how does it seem to go about coping? Observations of this kind can give us a rough idea of what the individual animal might be feeling. Once we relate our intuitions back to the remedies we should be able to come up with a few choices that may be appropriate. Reminding ourselves that the remedies can't do any harm is a comfort when we are forced to rely on educated guesswork.

Dosage for animals

Once we have made selections for our animals we need a way to give them the remedies. Dosage for animals, regardless of size and weight, is the same as for humans: four drops from a made-up treatment bottle, at least four times a day. But there are a few extra considerations to bear in mind. Some are to do with safety; others concern the practical difficulty of ensuring we give the right dose.

As far as safety goes, remember that there is a lot of brandy in a standard stock bottle. Some animals, including cats and birds, are extremely sensitive to alcohol. For this reason, we should avoid giving remedies to animals straight from the stock bottle. This doesn't apply, of course, if we are using an alcohol-free remedy.

The ideal way to give remedies to animals is to give four drops from a treatment bottle via a treat of some sort and repeat at least four times a day. This is preferable to giving drops direct from the built-in dropper because animals sometimes try to swallow or bite the glass. Even licking the pipette can cause a problem, as any contact between tongue and dropper will likely result in the treatment bottle contents becoming contaminated.

Some people find it convenient to use other delivery methods. A common approach is to add remedies to a water bowl or bucket or to food. A few owners stroke or drip the drops onto ears or paws, so that their animals take in the effects via the skin or by licking off the liquid. In terms of remedy effectiveness there is no problem with these methods. The drawback is that they can have unintended consequences. Cats in particular can be a problem. Smelling the remedy in their water or food they might refuse to drink or eat, which could have serious implications for their general health. Or you might find that your cat takes a violent dislike to having liquid placed on its ears – you could be creating fear and trauma instead of easing it. Be careful and observant if you try these methods and change tack if necessary.

Let's assume we have decided to put remedies into a water source. Perhaps we own a couple of ponies that live in a faraway field and we can't get out to see them four times a day. Our aim should be that, however little the animals drink in any one visit to the source, they will get at least the minimum dose each time: the equivalent of four drops from a treatment bottle. If we were making up a normal-sized bowl of water, two drops of each individual stock remedy (four of the crisis mix) would be sufficient. In effect it would be the same as making up a glass of water for a human being. But as the water source used by our ponies is larger, we will have to add more of each remedy to be confident that the minimum dose is being taken each time. The rule of thumb is to slightly more than double the dose: five drops of each individual stock remedy, ten drops of the crisis mix.

It doesn't matter if two or more animals share a dosed water bowl, since those that don't need the remedies will not be affected by them. Where two animals are being treated using different remedies we will have to find a way to dose them separately. Remember once again that if we are putting remedies in food or water we need to keep an eye on the animals to make sure they are happy taking remedies that way.

Easter bunnies

This story comes from a Bach practitioner in New York.

> Just after Easter I was in a local hardware store and saw a cage with two rabbits in it. They were left over from the holiday and nobody wanted them, so I took them home with me.
>
> I hadn't thought about my two dogs – West Highland terriers – and what their reaction would be to the new arrivals. Westies are hunters by instinct, so what they saw was something to chase and eat.
>
> I immediately made up a mix for the dogs. I put in Chicory for selfish possessiveness (the dogs love sitting

on my lap and did not like having to share), Walnut to help them get used to the change, Holly for their jealousy, Cherry Plum to help them keep their self-control and Willow for resentment.

They responded very quickly. Within three days dogs and rabbits had bonded and were bounding about the living room together, nuzzling each other happily. Now if I say to the dogs 'Where are your bunnies?' they will run to wherever the rabbits are.

Legal considerations when helping animals

In some parts of the world there are strict laws governing the provision of medical help to animals. In the UK, for example, acts of veterinary surgery can only be carried out by qualified veterinary surgeons, a law drawn up to protect animals from unlicensed practitioners who might put the health of animals at risk. Similar laws obtain in most parts of the US.

The exact status of Bach remedies under these laws is unclear; Dr Bach's system is never specifically mentioned. A judge might agree, if a case involving Bach remedies should ever come to court, that offering a flower remedy for a known fear should not be considered 'an act of veterinary surgery', since it is offering to treat an everyday emotional state and not a medical condition.

The good news is that in most countries people *are* allowed to treat their own animals and give emergency help to save a life. If you are not confident about the legal position where you live you should seek advice before you offer help to someone else's animal.

The Bach Centre instructs its practitioners to seek to work with animals under vet referral to ensure that any medical or veterinary condition is at all times under the care of a qualified person.

Remedies for plants

A family emigrating so the husband can find work, a dog frightened of strangers, a plant infested with parasites: all are under stress. Perhaps we should not be too surprised that a remedy for stress can help all three. Selecting specific remedies for plants can, however, be the most difficult challenge of all. The obvious remedies are the most used: the crisis combination when there has been a stressful event or illness, Crab Apple for attacks by fungus or insects, Walnut to help the plant adjust after re-potting or transplantation to a new garden.

We can go further, with a little imagination. We could start by looking at the shape of the plant and the way it holds itself. A plant that droops more than its neighbours might need Willow, Gentian, Gorse or Olive. Another that seems to resist everything and go on blooming might benefit from Oak or Agrimony. We can even try to put ourselves in the plant's position and select remedies based on how we think we would feel in those circumstances. This involves a lot of guesswork and a large dollop of assumption, of course, but because the remedies can't do any harm we can experiment without worrying about untoward consequences.

Dosage for plants is once again the same as for humans. If we knew the plant would absorb all the remedy we could make up a treatment bottle in the normal way and drip a four-drop dose into the middle of it. We usually, though, find it more convenient to give the remedies using a watering can or sprayer. Watering a single plant takes two drops of each stock remedy (four of the crisis mix) in a little water. When watering a larger area we would add five or so drops of each single remedy, or ten drops of the crisis mix, to each can of water. This allows a margin for error, because some of the remedy mix will not be taken up by the plant.

We would use the same strength dilution in a watering can if we were giving remedies to a tree. Best practice here is to water the ground that is sheltered by the branches. The roots of a tree cover roughly the same area, so this is an effective way to get remedy to each root. The remedies stay in the soil along with the water and will be absorbed gradually by the root system.

There is no need to water more than usual. However, if we prefer to give drops from a treatment bottle, to a houseplant, for example, we will need to repeat the dose at least four times a day.

8

What Do We Do if We Get Stuck?

Getting help and advice

For general help with dosage and understanding which remedy does what, The Bach Centre's website is a good place to start: www.bachcentre.com. It has links to sister sites in French, German, Italian and Spanish. There are full descriptions for each remedy and advice on selection as well as background information and a long list of frequently asked questions.

Dr Bach's aim was to create a simple system that anyone could use. 'It requires no science,' he once said, 'only a little knowledge and sympathy and understanding of human nature.' Nevertheless, sometimes our problems overwhelm us and working through them alone feels impossible. Maybe we just need some objective advice to help us define how we feel. If we would like a chance to discuss our feelings with an expert who can help identify our emotions and appropriate remedies, we should think about going to see a Bach practitioner.

How do I find a practitioner?

In many parts of the world anyone can set up as a practitioner or therapist. Some are well suited to the profession, others less so. As a potential client of a Bach flower therapist, you will want to ensure that you receive a good service. How should you go about finding a competent person?

One way is to find a local practitioner from the list on The Bach Centre's website. Practitioners registered with The Bach Centre – known as Bach Foundation Registered Practitioners or BFRPs – have followed an approved training programme that includes classroom teaching and written assessments. BFRPs agree to abide by a strict code of practice, which enforces acceptable standards of professional behaviour.

There are BFRPs all over the world and more are trained every year. Many offer telephone consultations to clients who live a long distance away. A few can arrange simple consultations by email as well.

Another starting point is to ask your local health food shop or pharmacy whether they can suggest a reliable local person. This can be a fruitful approach because local shops often know local practitioners pretty well, and they will be able to give you some informal advice on the person who will be best suited to you.

You could also contact one of the general registers of complementary therapists to see if they have any Bach practitioners on their books. Umbrella registers tend to be national rather than international in scope, so Google is the best way to find who is active in your country and who has the best reputation.

Contacting a practitioner

When you get in touch with a practitioner for the first time there are a few questions you should ask so as to be sure you know what kind of service you will receive.

- How much will the consultation cost? And what exactly does the charge include? Most practitioners will make an hourly charge that may or may not include the cost of a mixed treatment bottle. You might be asked to pay up front for a follow-up session (usually about 40 minutes) where the initial selection of remedies can be reviewed.

- How will remedies be selected? Traditional Bach practitioners (including all those on The Bach Centre's register) listen to how you feel and make recommendations on that basis. Other types of practitioner may select remedies by muscle testing, dowsing or other techniques.

- Does the practitioner follow a code of practice, ethics or conduct and/or belong to a professional body? It is important to know what standards are being worked to, and to whom you can complain if you feel you have not been treated well.

There are many good practitioners working with the remedies, so you should find somebody without too much difficulty. Whether you stick with the classic approach of a BFRP or prefer to see somebody who works in a different way, the important thing is to find out what is being offered so you can make an informed choice.

What happens during a consultation?

Dr Bach taught that a consultation should be a straightforward affair and reflect the simplicity of the therapy. The classic practitioner will start by asking you how much you know about the remedies and will tell you a little more about the system if that seems appropriate. Then she will ask why you have come and what you are having trouble with. The aim will be to find out how you feel about your current situation. As far as possible the practitioner will avoid putting words into your mouth so that you can describe your emotions in your way

There is no reason to be embarrassed about discussing your feelings. All the remedies reflect normal human emotions and, like everyone else, the practitioner will have gone through every negative state at some time or other. Nevertheless, if you find you need something at the start to settle you down, just ask the practitioner. Most will be happy to give you a remedy to deal with any immediate nerves.

The practitioner will aim to listen more than she talks, and if she does ask questions they will be aimed at finding out what unhappiness, stress or sadness actually feels like to you. She may ask about your reactions to everyday situations, or even to hypothetical scenarios, in order to ascertain the type remedy you might need.

Most first consultations last about an hour. Towards the end of this time the practitioner will sum up what she has understood, giving you a chance to correct any misunderstandings. She will then go through the remedies she thinks might apply, explaining her reasons for each selection. This gives you an opportunity to say if you don't agree with a choice.

Finally, she will mix up a treatment bottle for you, or perhaps invite you to do this yourself, or give you the address of a pharmacy that will mix up the bottle for you.

Arrangements for a follow-up visit might be made there and then, or you might be invited to phone in when you are ready to make a further appointment. Most follow-up visits will be arranged for two or three weeks after the first consultation, as this is the period that the treatment bottle will last.

How many consultations will I need?

There is no hard and fast rule as to how many consultations you will need. Classic Bach practitioners will encourage you to select remedies for yourself as soon as you feel able to do so. They will be aware that this is a self-help therapy and will encourage you to use it as such, rather than building up dependency on a practitioner. We often say at The Bach Centre that the best practitioners are the ones who lose all their clients and are happy to do so.

FINDING OUT MORE

Further reading

These books will give you a good grounding in the Bach remedies. They cover everything from the history of the system to its everyday application.

- Bach, E. (2009) *Heal Thyself.* Wallingford: The Bach Centre. A companion to *The Twelve Healers and Other Remedies,* this is Dr Bach's personal account of his philosophy of healing. The recommended edition is available for free from: www.bachcentre.com.

- Bach, E. (2011) *The Twelve Healers and Other Remedies – The Definitive Edition.* Wallingford: The Bach Centre. Dr Bach's final word on his discoveries includes the classic remedy descriptions. There are many editions of this book. The definitive edition was published to coincide with the 125th anniversary of Dr Bach's birth, and includes all the 1941 text, along with footnotes and a new introduction. It is available for free (and in multiple languages) from: www. bachcentre.com.

- Howard, J. and Ramsell, J. (eds) (1990) *The Original Writings of Edward Bach.* Saffron Walden: The C.W. Daniel Co. Dr Bach's earlier writings are essential reading for the serious student.

- Ramsell Howard, J. (2004) *Growing Up with Bach Flower Remedies.* London: Vermilion. This book explores how the remedies can be used to help children from birth to adolescence.

- Ramsell Howard, J. (2005) *Bach Flower Remedies for Women*. London: Vermilion. A complete guide showing how the remedies can apply to many common life situations that confront women.

- Weeks, N. (1940) *The Medical Discoveries of Edward Bach, Physician*. Saffron Walden: The C.W. Daniel Co. The most reliable work on the history of Dr Bach's life and discoveries, written by his assistant.

I would of course also recommend my own writings on the remedies, and in particular *The Bach Remedies Workbook* (an interactive text book), *Bloom* (which focuses on flower remedies and self-development), *Teach Yourself Bach Flower Remedies*, *Bach Flower Remedies for Men*, *Bach Flower Remedies for Animals* and *Emotional Healing for Cats* (both with Judy Ramsell Howard), and *Emotional Healing for Horses and Ponies* (with Judy Ramsell Howard and Heather Simpson). The horse book in particular is a key text for anybody interested in selecting remedies for animals.

Studying the remedies

Dr Bach's dream was to have remedies in every home, and to give the power of healing to anybody and everybody who wanted it. His is a simple system, so with what you have learned from this book – let alone what you can get from the other books listed – you have enough to start choosing remedies for yourself, your family and your friends.

For many of us, though, the remedies become a passion and a way of life. We want to learn more. We want to discuss them and debate them. We want to gain experience and hear other points of view.

There are courses and seminars and workshops on the Bach remedies all over the world. Any list printed here would quickly go out of date, so the best place to start looking for courses is once again The Bach Centre's website. The core Bach Centre-approved courses listed there – which run in 40 countries around the world – teach the classic approach and can take you from beginner all the way up to Bach Foundation Registered Practitioner level. In addition the website has links to informal events run by independent teachers. These include local two-hour meetings where anyone can go along and 'talk Bach' with other enthusiasts.

To find out more go to: www.bachcentre.com/learn.

Where to get your remedies

There are several companies making the 38 remedies in Dr Bach's system. The longest established brand, which traces its heritage via The Bach Centre to Dr Bach himself, is made and distributed by Nelsons (www.nelsons.net). Other makers in the UK include Healing Herbs and Ainsworths; and there are remedy makers in many other countries, some of them small operations that come and go quite quickly.

It is not difficult in the days of the internet to find remedies for sale online and they can normally be shipped to wherever you happen to live. Whether you shop online or go to your local health shop, however, I would advise that you stick with the better-known brands. Making remedies is easy, but it's not unknown for an inexperienced maker to inadvertently use the wrong plant. The degree of dilution means you are unlikely to be harmed by a flower remedy, even one that has been made badly. Better though to take a good remedy and experience for yourself how gentle and effective and wonderful this system can be.